To

Marvin

An Esteamed colleague

Morris

ATTACHMENT AND PSYCHOANALYSIS

Intersections: Psychoanalysis and Psychological Science

Elliot L. Jurist, Series Editor

While psychoanalysis rests on a foundation of theory and clinical knowledge, the time is now right to embrace research and to explore and deepen links to other fields. Books in this series bridge science and practice and elucidate the relationship between them, highlighting empirical findings and their impact on treatment and presenting substantive clinical work that might inspire and direct research. The aim of the series is to show that psychoanalysis is too compelling to be of interest only to psychoanalysts.

ATTACHMENT AND PSYCHOANALYSIS

Theory, Research, and Clinical Implications

MORRIS N. EAGLE

THE GUILFORD PRESS
New York   London

Library of Congress Cataloging-in-Publication Data

Eagle, Morris N.
  Attachment and psychoanalysis : theory, research, and clinical implications /
Morris N. Eagle.
     pages cm.—(Intersections : psychoanalysis and psychological science)
  Includes bibliographical references and index.
  ISBN 978-1-4625-0840-2 (hardback : acid-free paper)
  1. Attachment behavior. 2. Psychoanalysis. 3. Psychotherapy. I. Title.
  RC455.4.A84E24 2013
  152.4′1—dc23
                                                          2012041740

To Rita

About the Author

Morris N. Eagle, PhD, ABPP, is Distinguished Educator in Residence at California Lutheran University, Thousand Oaks, California, and Professor Emeritus at the Derner Institute for Advanced Psychological Studies, Adelphi University, Garden City, New York. His publications include the books *From Classical to Contemporary Psychoanalysis: A Critique and Integration, Recent Developments in Psychoanalysis: A Critical Evaluation,* and *The Interface of Psychoanalysis and Psychology* (coedited with James W. Barron and David L. Wolitzky). He is also the author of more than 100 journal articles and 100 presentations. Dr. Eagle is a past president of the Division of Psychoanalysis (Division 39) of the American Psychological Association, a recipient of the 2009 Sigourney Award for distinguished contributions to the field of psychoanalysis, and cofounder, along with Everett Waters and Gary Cox-Steiner, of the New York Attachment Consortium.

Preface

This book deals with the relationship between attachment theory and psychoanalysis. Despite the fact that the origins of attachment theory largely lie in psychoanalysis, as Peter Fonagy (2001) notes, there has been "bad blood" between the two disciplines. One central aim of this book is to contribute to reducing these ill feelings and to replace this state of affairs with a deeper level of understanding, and perhaps even point to possible areas of partial integration.

One of the suggestions made by Elliot Jurist, who served as a very helpful reviewer of a draft of the manuscript, was to use the preface to communicate in my own voice how I was drawn to attachment theory. I had not thought of discussing my personal experience and worried that it might seem too egocentric. However, the more I thought about it, the more it seemed to me not at all a bad idea—particularly if it succeeded in conveying a picture of the kinds of experiences that would make it natural for someone with a psychoanalytic background to become vitally interested in attachment theory.

I became interested in attachment theory and research many years ago after reading the first two volumes of John Bowlby's trilogy on attachment. I think a more serious interest began to develop around the time that I reviewed Volume 3 for the *Review of Psychoanalytic Books* (Eagle, 1982). After reading all three volumes, I felt that attachment theory constituted an extremely important contribution to advancing an understanding of a core aspect of human (and animal) nature, namely, the nature of our attachment to others. Furthermore, I felt that not only the content but also the *form*, so to speak, of Bowlby's contributions were very important. That is to say, Bowlby appealed to data (from relevant disciplines) rather than to authority or "clinical experience" in his theorizing. His language was straightforward and accessible and referred to ordinary psychological processes about which we know a great deal rather than to esoteric entities far removed from experience and behavior. Also, despite being subject to attacks and misunderstandings from the psychoanalytic establishment, he confidently forged ahead with his work. As I stated in the last sentence of my review of Volume 3, he was a man of one piece. This impression of Bowlby, based on his writing, was confirmed when I met him during his visit to the Toronto Psychoanalytic Institute in the 1980s.

My own background and training drew me not only to attachment theory and research, but to any research and theoretical developments that linked psychoanalytic theory to theories and findings from psychology and other relevant disciplines. I was fortunate enough to have been admitted to a remarkable master's program in clinical psychology at the City College of New York established by Joseph E. Barmack after his stint as a research candidate at the New York Psychoanalytic Institute. The heavily psychoanalytic courses offered were given by David Beres, Ernst Kris, Katherine Wolf, Ruth Monroe, Bela Mittelmann, and Roy Schafer, among others. The program also included a year-long course by Kurt Goldstein on his classic book *The Organism* and an inspiring course by Daniel Lehrman on animal behavior. The five of us who were admitted to the program lived and breathed psychoanalysis.

My passion for psychoanalysis was nurtured further at the doctoral clinical program at New York University and by my appointment as a predoctoral Fellow (and later as Research Assistant Professor) at the University's Research Center for Mental Health, codirected by George S. Klein and Robert Holt, whose mandate was to carry out research that, directly or indirectly, was relevant to psychoanalytic propositions. The Center was an extraordinarily exciting and stimulating place, abuzz with the latest research and thinking presented by invited speakers and staff, including David Wolitzky, Fred Pine, Leo Goldberger, and Donald Spence. We were also fortunate to have David Rapaport, Merton Gill, and Hartvig Dahl as visiting faculty. The Center's unifying motifs were research relevant to psychoanalytic propositions, as noted, and bringing to bear findings from other relevant disciplines on psychoanalytic theorizing.

My main research activities during my tenure there involved the role of intention and attention in learning, memory, and perception. The research I conducted with colleagues on, for example, incidental learning, was published in nonpsychoanalytic journals, including the *American Journal of*

Psychology (Eagle, 1967; Eagle & Mulliken, 1974), the *Journal of Experimental Psychology* (Cramer & Eagle, 1972; Eagle & Leiter, 1964; Stoff & Eagle, 1971), and the *Journal of Verbal Learning and Verbal Behavior* (Eagle & Ortof, 1967). This was also the case for other research on perception, including "subliminal perception," that was published in *Nature* (Eagle & Hill, 1969), *Science* (Eagle, Wolitzky, & Klein, 1966), and the *Journal of Nervous and Mental Disease* (Eagle, 1962). Although certainly not evident, much of this research *was* stimulated by psychoanalytic ideas (particularly Rapaport's) on attention.

The indirect links to psychoanalytic theory and the publication of articles in nonpsychoanalytic journals—at the time psychoanalytic journals did not publish empirical research—also characterized virtually all the Center's work. Although none of the research, conducted before Bowlby's trilogy was published, had to do with attachment theory, the direction of our attention outward to findings in other disciplines and the strong valuing of empirical research paved the way for my eventual interest in attachment theory and research. One could not find a better exemplar of a body of work that combined so well a focus on matters of great relevance for psychoanalysis and the valuing of empirical research.

In 1993, I presented a paper on attachment and psychoanalysis at a conference on psychotherapy and attachment sponsored by the British Psychological Society and the Royal College of Psychiatrists in London. There I met Kim Bartholomew, a co-presenter, and Richard Bowlby, Susan Orbach, and Joseph Schwartz, the conference organizers. The resulting article was published in the *British Journal of Medical Psychology* (Eagle, 1995).

Another major conference on attachment was held in Toronto in 1994, at which I presented a paper entitled "The Developmental Perspectives of Attachment and Psychoanalytic Theories," which appeared as a chapter in a book edited by Susan Goldberg, Roy Muir, and John Kerr (1995) entitled *Attachment Theory: Social, Developmental, and Clinical Perspectives*. Other presenters included Arietta Slade, Peter Fonagy, Roy Muir, and Susan Goldberg. In 1996, I contributed a chapter on "Attachment Research and Psychoanalytic Theory" to the book *Psychoanalytic Perspectives on Developmental Psychology*, edited by Joseph Masling and Robert Bornstein (Eagle, 1996).

My large-scale involvement with attachment theory and research was hugely facilitated by the support of the Mental Health Foundation, headed by Jenny and Gary Cox-Steiner, two lovely, incredibly generous, and highly intelligent and altruistic people, who wanted to contribute to the furthering of mental health research in children and their caregivers. The Mental Health Foundation provided grants to doctoral students at Adelphi University, Stony Brook University, City University of New York, and Yale

University whose dissertations were in the area of attachment. In addition, the Foundation supported my work, and sponsored attachment conferences and the establishment of the New York Attachment Consortium at Adelphi University, which was originally led by Gary Cox-Steiner, Everett Waters, and me. After I left Adelphi in 2004, Gary Cox-Steiner and Everett Waters remained as directors of the Consortium.

In 2000, with the support of the Mental Health Foundation, Gary Cox-Steiner, Arietta Slade, and I organized a major 2-day conference on "Attachment: Current Developments in Research, Theory, and Application." The participants, besides me, included Peter Fonagy, Erik Hesse, Mary Main, Beatrice Beebe, Judith Crowell, Myron Hofer, June Sroufe, Alan Sroufe, Mary Target, Jay Belsky, Karlin Lyons-Ruth, and Arietta Slade. The articles appeared in a special volume of the *Journal of Infant and Adolescent Psychotherapy* (Eagle & Cox-Steiner, 2001) that I and Gary Cox-Steiner edited.

During the next few years, a number of conferences were all organized by Gary Cox-Steiner and Everett Waters for the New York Attachment Consortium with the support of the Mental Health Foundation. A 2003 conference brought together leading attachment researchers and theorists from both the social psychology self-report approach and the developmental psychology Adult Attachment Interview approach to the measurement of adult attachment. The participants included me, Phil Shaver, Mario Mikulincer, Ken Levy, Everett Waters, and Alan Sroufe, among others. Two smaller-scale conferences were held at Adelphi University. The theme of the first one in 2005 was "Attachment and Sexuality" and was organized around my paper on that topic. The participants included Diana Diamond, Geoff Goodman, Ken Levy, Doris Silverman, Howard Steele, Jerome Wakefield, and Everett Waters. A version of my paper was published in 2007 as a chapter in the book *Attachment and Sexuality*, edited by Diana Diamond, Sidney Blatt, and Joseph Lichtenberg (Eagle, 2007).

The theme of the second and final conference in 2006 was "Adult Psychotherapy: The Perspectives of Attachment Theory and Psychoanalysis." It was organized around my 2006 commentary on five articles on attachment-oriented therapeutic interventions published in the *Journal of Consulting and Clinical Psychology*. The participants at the conference were Joseph Lichtenberg, Doris Silverman, Joanne Davila, Geoff Goodman, Doris Silverman, Miriam Steele, and Everett Waters.

The plan of the book is as follows: The first four chapters present an overview of attachment theory and research as a foundation for a subsequent discussion of the relationship between attachment theory and research and psychoanalysis. After reading Chapters 1–4, the reader will be reasonably familiar with the fundamental issues of attachment theory and with some key research findings relevant to these issues.

Chapters 5 and 6 review the main points of divergence between attachment theory and early and later psychoanalytic theories. Any attempt at integration between attachment theory and psychoanalysis needs to take into account these areas of divergence.

The next four chapters, 7–10, are devoted to central aspects of human behavior: sexuality, aggression, and psychopathology from the perspectives of attachment theory and psychoanalysis. The implications of attachment theory and research for clinical interventions are then discussed in Chapter 11.

The concluding chapter, Chapter 12, takes up points of convergence between attachment and psychoanalytic theories and areas of potential integration between the two perspectives.

I hope that the book will clarify important issues and facilitate a greater degree of integration between attachment theory and psychoanalysis.

Acknowledgments

I am grateful to Elliot Jurist for his comments and suggestions. I am also extremely grateful to Everett Waters, not only for his collaboration on the first three chapters, but also for his willingness to share his extensive knowledge and judgment on all matters related to attachment theory and research. I want to thank my research assistant, Miranda Sager, who tracked down endless references and who, miraculously, was able to decipher and type my handwritten material. And last—and certainly not least, but rather most—I especially want to express my appreciation and gratitude to my wife, Rita, who went over every chapter with a fine-tooth comb, correcting inconsistencies and lack of clarity, offering new ideas, and, above all, contributing mightily to the coherent organization of the material.

Contents

CHAPTER 1

Historical Introduction

In collaboration with Everett Waters

The first sentence of Fonagy's (2001) book *Attachment Theory and Psychoanalysis* reads: "There is bad blood between psychoanalysis and attachment theory" (p. 1). This is less true today than it has been in the past. However, it remains the case that there is a continuing tension between psychoanalysis and attachment theory. This is so for a number of reasons, including both the impact of the history of their relationship and an incompatibility, or at least a divergence, between their respective approaches to how one comes to understand human nature and the individual.

I begin with a brief account of the history of the relationship between attachment theory and psychoanalysis. Insofar as attachment theory began as a reaction against and intended corrective to certain aspects of Freudian and Kleinian theory, tracing its relationship to psychoanalysis helps one understand some aspects of the conceptual origins of attachment theory. My focus in this chapter is on conceptual, theoretical, and clinical issues rather than on straightforward historical and biographical details. The

Everett Waters, PhD, is Professor of Psychology at the Stony Brook University and a founding member of the New York Attachment Consortium. His extensive publications include the classic volume *Patterns of Attachment* (coauthored with Mary Ainsworth and colleagues) and two *Monographs of the Society for Research in Child Development*.

latter is available from a number of excellent sources (e.g., Karen, 1994; Newcombe & Lerner, 1982; van der Horst, 2011).

I include a few highly pertinent biographical details in order to set the stage. One such detail is the fact that Bowlby, the father of attachment theory, was trained as a psychoanalyst—at the British Psychoanalytic Society—and viewed himself as an analyst throughout his life. A second important biographical detail concerns Bowlby's early clinical experiences and influences. The precursors of Bowlby's work on attachment theory began at age 21 during his work in a home for maladjusted boys. Early in his career (1928–1929), Bowlby temporarily abandoned his medical education to do volunteer work at two progressive education residential institutions for disturbed children, including a 6-month stint at one of them (Priority Gate School). These experiences had a profound impact on Bowlby, who comments with regard to the time spent at the second institution, "Everything stemmed from that six months" (as cited in Karen, 1994, p. 33). As van der Horst (2011) documents, "progressive" schools at the time, including Priority Gate School, were strongly influenced by psychoanalytic ideas, including the central idea that early deprivation of love was the primary source of later mental problems (Lane, 1928).

In 1936, Bowlby took a half-time job at the London Child Guidance Clinic, where he worked for 3 years. It was these and related experiences that led Bowlby to emphasize the disruption of the early mother–child relationship as a key factor in later psychopathology. Bowlby's views were further supported by the work of Robertson (1962) on separation of young children from parents due to hospitalization and later by the research of Heinicke (1956) and Heinicke and Westheimer (1966). Bowlby's great interest in the effects of early maternal deprivation on the psychological development of the child led to work for the World Health Organization, culminating in a monograph entitled *Maternal Care and Mental Health* followed by *Child Care and the Growth of Love*, which was published in 1952 and sold a huge number of copies.

Bowlby's thinking during this period of time marked the pre-attachment theory phase of Bowlby's writings, which, of course, set the stage for the later explicitly formulated theory. During this phase, Bowlby's main focus was on the effects of maternal care—for example, separation, mistreatment, the presence or absence of love—on development. His early professional experiences with maladjusted children were very likely different from those of most psychoanalysts and were bound to influence his thinking. The people who most influenced Bowlby early in his career were not analysts, but social workers, among them James Robertson, Molly Lowden, and Nance Fairbairn at the London Child Guidance Clinic, and

John Alford, who though not trained as a social worker, essentially functioned as one in one of the residential institutions at which Bowlby volunteered. It was Alford who encouraged Bowlby to seek psychoanalytic training, which he began at the age of 22 in 1929. The social work emphasis on the actual familial and social circumstances of the child's life—an emphasis so different from the near exclusive psychoanalytic concern with intrapsychic factors—undoubtedly had a strong impact on his theorizing. There is the well-known account of Klein as Bowlby's supervisor refusing to allow him to have contact with the mother of a child in treatment.

In a recent paper, van der Horst (2011) notes the major influence on Bowlby of the "English" school of psychiatry located mainly at the Tavistock Clinic and led by Ian Suttie. As van der Horst demonstrates, Suttie's (1935/1988) classic *The Origins of Love and Hate* had a great deal of influence on Bowlby's ideas. Both Suttie and Bowlby were also influenced by the Hungarian School that included Imre Hermann, Michael and Alice Balint, and, above all, Sandor Ferenczi (see Bacciagaluppi, 1994). In striking similarity to Bowlby's ideas, Suttie wrote that the infant's "love of mother is primal" (p. 31) and expressed skepticism of the claim that the "attachment-to-mother is merely the sum of the infantile bodily needs and satisfaction" (p. 16).[1]

Another important influence on Bowlby's thinking was the work of ethologists such as Konrad Lorenz (e.g., 1935) and R. A. Hinde (e.g., 1982). Lorenz's work on imprinting suggested to Bowlby the idea that infants of different species are genetically predisposed to form a bond with, that is, to become attached to, a figure with whom they come into contact early in life. Furthermore, the imprinting phenomenon suggested that the attachment bond did not depend on being fed by this early figure—a view contrary to prevailing theory. Bowlby was also aware of Harlow's (1958) work demonstrating the relative roles of food and "contact comfort" in the infant monkey's attachment to its surrogate mother.

The imprinting phenomenon also constituted evidence of the role of evolution in shaping a species' learning propensities, an important consideration in attachment theory. It is important to note that Bowlby's interest in ethology was but one expression of the deep and abiding influence of evolutionary theory on his thinking. Indeed, later in his life, Bowlby wrote a biography of Darwin, undoubtedly one of his heroes. Bowlby recognized the obvious adaptive value of imprinting and thought it very likely that something like imprinting had been selected for in mammalian species. Of

---

[1]Interestingly, in a recent paper, Clarke (2011) traces the influence of Suttie's ideas on Fairbairn's object relations theory.

course, this mammalian analogue of imprinting was nothing less than the attachment instinctual system.

A second important influence on Bowlby's thinking was the body of ideas generated by information theory and cybernetic systems theory, precursors to the cognitive revolution in psychology. These ideas played a role not in influencing Bowlby's positing of a selected for instinctual attachment system—information theory was not relevant to that issue—but in formulating how the system operated. Bowlby wanted to replace the Freudian account of instinctual drives in terms of buildup and discharge of energy with an account of instinctual systems in terms of feedback and control. One should also note the somewhat circumscribed influence of the cognitive psychologist Craik and of Piaget's concepts of schemas and assimilation on Bowlby's later concept of "working model."

The last and certainly not least influences on Bowlby were the Freudian and Kleinian psychoanalytic theories to which he was exposed. Bowlby studied psychology at Cambridge in 1925 where his tutor in the natural sciences was E. D. Adrian, a world-renowned neuroscientist who was very interested in Freudian theory and even published a paper in 1946 in the *International Journal of Psychoanalysis*. Van der Horst speculates that Bowlby might have discussed Freudian theory with Adrian. What we do know, however, is that Bowlby read Freud's *Introductory Lectures on Psychoanalysis* and later ranked it as among the 11 most important books he had ever read (van der Horst, 2011).

The influence of psychoanalytic theory on Bowlby's thinking was important in both a "positive" and "negative" sense. Bowlby found much that he believed to be mistaken in psychoanalytic theory. However, it is easy to lose sight of the positive influences of psychoanalysis on Bowlby because they are often taken for granted. That is, as noted, Bowlby viewed himself as an analyst throughout his life, and his goal in developing attachment theory was not to set it up as an alternative to psychoanalysis, but as a corrective to what he believed to be certain major errors and defects of psychoanalytic theory. He also wanted to preserve the insights provided by psychoanalysis, for example, the critical importance of early experiences for later development (Waters, 2009). His intention was to reform psychoanalysis and align it with current scientific theories and findings—and thereby preserve it and endow it with a new vitality—rather than destroy or overthrow it.

In recounting the history of attachment theory, one confronts unattractive aspects of the history of psychoanalysis. Bowlby was treated as a pariah by the British Psychoanalytic Society. Rather than making a serious effort to understand the fundamentals of attachment theory, many in the psychoanalytic community summarily dismissed it, often because it was deemed nonpsychoanalytic—a standard criticism directed against "revisionist" theories.

As Fonagy (2001) observes, "Analysts make dismissive comments about [Bowlby's] work yet feel no obligation to read it" (p. 2). Some examples of rather mindless criticisms include Isaacs's comment that "an infant can't follow its mother; it isn't a duckling" (cited in Scarf, 1976, p. 151) and Segal's (cited in a 1989 interview with Karen, 1994) quote from Ogden Nash: "What's the use to psychoanalyze a goose." As Karen (1994) points out, Bowlby's (1960) paper in the *Psychoanalytic Study of the Child* was followed by three rejoinders by Anna Freud, Max Schur, and René Spitz that appeared "without informing Bowlby or giving him a chance to reply" (Karen, p. 113). Furthermore, according to Karen, "in the annual's fifteen years of publication no replies like this had ever appeared before and none have appeared in the thirty years since" (p. 114).

Frequent critiques levied against attachment theory were often based, not on empirical data, including clinical data, but on the criticism that certain of its tenets violated or did not conform to presumed fundamental psychoanalytic assumptions and formulations—without raising questions regarding the empirical support for these assumptions and formulations. As we see in later chapters, in certain psychoanalytic circles, the attitude that attachment theory, the phenomena it deals with, and the methods by which it deals with them are not properly part of psychoanalysis continues pretty much to the present day. Fortunately, this attitude has been balanced during the last 15 or 20 years by a number of developments that have made psychoanalysis more hospitable to attachment theory and research. The more important of these developments include critiques of Freudian drive theory, a relative deemphasis on sexual and aggressive wishes and a concomitant increased emphasis on relational motives and on interactional processes, and the emergence of a cadre of psychoanalytic researchers who, given their research orientation, are more sympathetic and open to attachment theory and research.

The last few years have seen the lessening of the "bad blood between psychoanalysis and attachment theory" to which Fonagy (2001, p. 1) refers. One can observe the eagerness of a number of psychoanalytic institutes to include a few lectures on attachment theory and research in their curriculum, even if they are generally not ready to offer a full course on the topic. One finds papers by leading attachment theorists and researchers, such as A few years ago, I attended an invited lecture given by a leading attachment theorist and researcher, Everett Waters (2009), at the New York Psychoanalytic Institute. And recently, Phillip Shaver (2011), a leading attachment researcher, was invited to present his work at a panel of the spring meetings of the American Psychoanalytic Association.

Nonetheless, tension between psychoanalysis and attachment theory remains and is likely to continue. This is quite understandable given their different attitudes and orientations and given the fact that analysts whose main professional activity is clinical work often do not find direct relevance to their work in the general findings of attachment research. However, a greater degree of mutual acceptance and greater contact between the two disciplines make this an opportune time to take another look at their relationship.

CHAPTER 2

Core Tenets of Attachment Theory

In collaboration with Everett Waters

ATTACHMENT AS AN AUTONOMOUS BEHAVIORAL SYSTEM

The core tenets of attachment theory can be identified at different levels of abstraction and generalization. There are essential background assumptions; core tenets that are primary and fundamental; and formulations that are important but that can be viewed as secondary—that is, if not supported, would not do fatal damage to the theory. At the most general level, a core tenet of attachment theory is the assumption that in the course of evolution, an autonomous attachment behavioral system had been selected for in a wide range of species, including humans, due to the adaptive advantage it confers on the individual. A primary adaptive advantage conferred by the attachment system is the enhancement of safety and therefore survival. Bowlby (1969/1982) specifically identified protection from predators—through the infant's inborn tendency to seek proximity to the caregiver. The presence of this tendency immediately after birth and its appearance across a wide range of species points to its selected-for evolutionary basis.

Other components of the attachment behavioral system include vocalization (e.g., crying), smiling, clinging, sucking, and later locomotion, all of which serve to bring about or maintain proximity to the caregiver. To be noted here is that "signals" such as crying or smiling are effective in

7

achieving proximity only in the context of a reciprocal caregiving system. That is, sucking, smiling, and vocalizing are likely to achieve proximity to an adult who responds to the cues by engaging in caregiving behavior. For example, there is nothing as effective as an infant's smile (as well as other neotenous features) to elicit loving, affectionate, and caregiving responses in an adult. One can think of the infant's smile as but one aspect of the general attraction that the young have for adults. One simply needs to observe the response of adults to kittens or puppies to see this tendency in action. One can think of the adult's potential caregiving behavior as the environmental niche to which the attachment system is adapted.

I refer to attachment as an *autonomous* behavioral system to make clear Bowlby's insistence that the infant's attachment to the caregiver is not reducible to or secondarily derived from other experiences and gratification of presumably more primary instinctual systems such as the hunger drive. Bowlby's positing of an autonomous attachment behavioral system represented a clear point of divergence from Freudian theory. In this regard, Bowlby's theorizing was quite congruent with Fairbairn's (1952) claim that "libido is primarily object-seeking (rather than pleasure-seeking as in the classic theory" (p. 82). As Fonagy (2001) observes, however, there is a subtle distinction between Bowlby's emphasis on the goal of the desired degree of proximity to the mother—a physical state—and Fairbairn's emphasis on the object (i.e., mother) itself as the goal.

Another general assumption of attachment theory, one that it shares with psychoanalysis, is that early experiences play a determinative role in psychological development. However, the early experiences emphasized by Bowlby have to do with the child's interactions with his or her caregiver and in particular, with such experiences as continuity of care versus disruption and sensitive caring versus neglect. Finally, another general background assumption of attachment theory is that intimate attachments are at the center of one's emotional life from infancy to adulthood to old age. Let me turn now to more specific core tenets of attachment theory.

LINKS BETWEEN THE ATTACHMENT AND FEAR SYSTEMS

An intimate link exists between the attachment and fear systems. Comforting a frightened child is one of the caregiver's primary functions. The experience of fear in response to cues of danger, such as unfamiliarity, sudden noise, darkness, and being alone, activates the attachment system which behaviorly, means seeking proximity to the caregiver. When proximity is achieved, fear is reduced. That is, the child is comforted and soothed and the attachment system is deactivated. The ability of the caregiver to comfort the child who is experiencing fear speaks to one of the primary functions of the attachment figure: the safe haven function. This function is clearly illustrated in Harlow's (1958) paper "The Nature of Love." When a toy "monster" is placed in the room, the infant monkey cowers in the corner with fear. However, when the terry cloth surrogate mother is introduced into the room, the monkey clings to it and is now suddenly endowed with courage and even swats at the "monster." A previously fear-inducing object is now far less frightening. Note that the functional relationship I have described operates as an affect-regulating negative feedback system—much like the way a thermostat operates: fear → attachment system activated → proximity to caregiver sought → achieved proximity reduces fear → attachment system deactivated.

One should note that it is not just fear that activates the attachment system, but also forms of distress (such as being ill or in pain). As a brief anticipation of a later discussion, imagine the consequences of a breakdown in this negative feedback system. For example, what is likely to happen if the safe haven function of the attachment figure does not operate adequately?

I have described the function of proximity to the attachment figure in reducing fear that the child experiences, taking for granted that there are what Bowlby (1973) referred to as "natural" cues to danger (e.g., sudden noise) that elicit fear in any child. However, the degree of fear experienced or perhaps even whether fear is experienced in the first place is strongly influenced by whether the attachment figure is present, as well as the behavior of the attachment figure. Thus, with regard to the first point, if they could experience the toy "monster" while clinging to the surrogate mother, Harlow's monkeys would undoubtedly have experienced less fear. Perhaps it is too subtle a point, but I am making a distinction between the function of the attachment figure in comforting and soothing the child who has already experienced fear and the function of the attachment figure in rendering fear-inducing situations and stimuli that would otherwise elicit strong fear less fearful.

A good historical illustration of this latter function is seen in the reports that, despite the obvious extreme realistic danger during the London Blitz of World War II, the degree of fear experienced by the children who experienced the bombings varied with parental availability and responses. That is, the degree of fear experienced by the child varied with how much fear the caregivers expressed. This influence seems different from the safe haven function when the latter is understood as soothing and comforting fear that has already been elicited.

My intuition is that there is a meaningful clinical distinction between the role of the attachment figure in providing comforting and soothing in response to fear that has been elicited and the role of the attachment figure in influencing degree of fear or whether fear is experienced in the first place. Although it is the former that is mainly emphasized, I think that the latter is also an important function of the attachment figure and plays a role in the secure base function of the attachment figure.

LINKS BETWEEN THE ATTACHMENT AND EXPLORATORY SYSTEMS

The attachment and exploratory systems are as intertwined as the attachment and fear systems, but in a different way. Whereas fear activates the attachment system, exploratory activity is more likely to occur when the attachment system is deactivated. Another way to put this is to say that exploratory activity is highly unlikely when the infant's primary motive is to seek proximity to the caregiver, that is, when the attachment system is activated.[1] The goal or motive of seeking proximity to the caregiver when afraid or distressed in other ways is at odds with the goal or motive of exploring the world. They, so to speak, move the child in opposite directions. As Gullestad (2001) notes, "Without a secure base, the child constantly 'monitors' his caregivers. There is no freedom to play and to encounter the world" (p. 7).

What permits the attachment system to be relatively quiescent so that exploratory activity can occur is the actual and potential availability of the attachment figure. This speaks to the *secure base* function, another primary function of the attachment figure. All one need do to be convinced of the importance of the secure base function is to observe a toddler, say, playing in a sandbox with mother at some modest distance, say, talking to friends. Mother can easily see toddler and toddler can easily see mother, and all goes well. The exploratory-play system is in full swing, and the attachment system is nicely at rest—both made possible by the presence and the availability of mother. Now imagine what would happen if the toddler looked up from his or her play to find that mommy is not there, not to be seen. The play stops on a dime and is replaced by distress, searching, and

---

[1] Although the attachment literature commonly refers to activation and deactivation of the attachment system, Ainsworth et al. (1978) have noted that the attachment system needs to be continuously active in order to monitor relevant cues. It would perhaps be more accurate to refer to the relative dominance of exploratory or proximity-seeking behaviors. This issue also arises in viewing avoidant attachment in terms of deactivation and preoccupied attachment in terms of hyperactivation of the attachment system (see Chapter 3).

seeking proximity to mommy. The toddler's entire motivational hierarchy has been altered. Exploratory-play motives have been replaced by attachment motives. That is, the exploratory-play system has been deactivated, and the attachment system has been fully activated.

In all species studied—chicks, dogs, monkeys, and humans—the availability of the attachment figure increases the range of exploratory activity (Rajecki, Lamb, & Obmascher, 1978). In one study, simply having a photograph of mother in the room increased the range of toddlers' exploratory activity (Passman & Erck, 1977). In humans, one can study the effects not only of the physical availability, but also the attentional and emotional availability of the attachment figure. Thus, Sorce and Emde (1981) found that whereas mother's physical availability (mother is in the room reading a newspaper) facilitates the range and ease of the toddler's exploratory activity, her emotional and attentional availability (mother is not engaged in activity that requires her attention) does so even more.

The secure base function in facilitating exploratory activity has important ramifications for psychological and social development. In order for an infant and child to become a competent adult, he or she must acquire a range of skills and knowledge about the physical and social worlds. In most species, gross failures in the acquisition of such knowledge and skills threatens survival. The point here is that exploration is a vital behavioral system linked to survival in a long-term way. Hence, one can say that insofar as the secure base facilitates exploration, the attachment system contributes to survival not only in its more obvious and immediate function of enhancing safety (e.g., protection from predators), but also in its long-term function of making possible the acquisition of knowledge and skills necessary for adult functioning. Also, the long period of helplessness that characterizes the human species entails prolonged attachment with adult members of the species, which makes possible the acquisition of social knowledge and competence. Indeed, Fonagy et al. (1995) propose that an important function of the attachment system in humans is the development of an interpersonal interpretive mechanism, which permits one to function in a complex social world. In other words, one needs to be in a close long-term relationship with another in order to learn how to interpret social cues, a capacity necessary for successful social interaction.

Clearly, then, attachment is not simply a matter of feeling comforted and soothed, but also of such hard-headed considerations as competence and the development of skills. The attachment figure's emotional availability when the child is distressed (e.g., is ill), overly dependent, and not terribly competent, and the absence of availability when the child engages in exploratory and autonomous behavior do not constitute a recipe for optimal development. One can say that in such cases, even the attachment figure's safe haven function is partial and selective. That is, it is reserved for situations that do not involve exploratory and autonomous behavior. Further, as Marvin, Cooper, Hoffman, and Powell (2002) note, the security entails not only the caregiver's physical and emotional availability, but also encouraging and taking delight in the child's exploratory activity. It would not be very advantageous to the developing child if he or she experienced the attachment figure only in relation to her safe haven function and not at all in relation to her secure base function in facilitating exploration.[2]

Optimally, the safe haven and secure base functions of the attachment figure operate smoothly together in a way that Marvin et al. (2002) refer to as the "circle of security." The child's repeated experiences of the attachment figure as a safe haven when distressed results in the child's feeling of safety and "felt security" (Sroufe & Waters, 1977). That is, the child feels trust that the caregiver will be available should he or she feel distress and fear. This trusting expectation enables the child to take the risks that exploration and novelty often entail, which is another way of saying that the child now experiences the attachment figure as a secure base from which to explore the world. Exploration is now less fraught with anxiety because the child trusts that should danger arise he or she can turn to the attachment figure for safety.

Consider the example of the child going to school for the first time. This is a new and potentially anxiety-provoking situation, sometimes generating so-called school phobia. However, as Bowlby (1973) has pointed out, most often it is not the school the child is afraid of. Rather, the child is afraid that something will happen to mother and that she will not be available should the need for her arise. Thus, when operating optimally, the safe haven and secure base functions of the attachment figure are two sides of the same coin—hence, the term "circle of security."

I recall supervising a therapist who was treating a 9-year-old boy who was referred because of a school phobia. He was a remarkably open and insightful child and reported that he always worried about his mother after she dropped him off at school. He was concerned that some harm would befall her. On those days when his aunt rather than his mother took him

---

[2]Such a state of affairs brings to mind Masterson and Rinsley's (1975) proposal that the early history of individuals with borderline personality disorder is characterized by maternal emotional availability when the child is dependent and distressed and maternal emotional withdrawal when the child makes moves toward exploration and autonomy. From an attachment theory perspective, one can say that the attachment figure functions mainly as a safe haven and minimally as a secure base.

to school, the little boy was much less anxious at school. A creative teacher came up with the idea that the child be given a cell phone so that the child could make sure that his mother arrived home safely. The implementation of this idea went a long way toward reducing the child's anxiety. Much more, of course, can said about this case. But what is striking about it is the degree to which it follows the dynamics noted by Bowlby.

DISTAL FUNCTIONS AND PROXIMAL MOTIVES

Before continuing, it is important to note the distinction between *distal evolutionary functions and proximal causes and motives*. As we have seen, Bowlby (1969/1982) proposes that the infant's inborn tendency to seek proximity to the caregiver that has been selected for serves the distal evolutionary function of protection from predators and thereby enhances the likelihood of the infant's survival. This distal evolutionary function does not speak to the proximal causes or motives that account for proximity-seeking behavior. The infant does not seek proximity to the caregiver to be protected from predators. Rather, the infant's proximity-seeking behavior is likely to be motivated by such factors as seeking warmth, milk, and tactile stimulation.

The distinction between distal functions and proximal motives can be made clear by reference to sexual behavior. A distal function of sexual reproduction is that it enhances the individual's "inclusive fitness" (Trivers, 1971) and serves to propagate the species. However, the proximal motive for engaging in sexual intercourse is not to enhance inclusive fitness or to propagate the species but to experience pleasure.

We are not robots propelled by inborn tendencies serving distal functions. Rather, distal functions have an impact on behavior by influencing what is pleasurable and what is unpleasurable, what we want and do not want to do. Thus, whatever distal functions the attachment system serves, the role it plays in our lives have to do with such matters as "felt security," as feeling comforted when afraid, as feeling safe when exploring, and as feeling a strong emotional bond.

INTERNAL WORKING MODELS

In the above section, the language employed has been mainly an impersonal one of behaviors and activation and deactivation of behavioral systems. However, I have also referred to the child's *expectations* regarding the availability of the attachment figure, which implies *representations* of some kind. Bowlby (1973) proposed that the child's experiences and behaviors in relation to the attachment figure are undergirded by the representations formed on the basis of past experiences with the attachment figure. Following Craik (1943), a cognitive psychologist, and perhaps influenced by the Piagetian concepts of schemas, assimilation and accommodation, Bowlby proposed the idea that the infant and child developed *internal working models* regarding the attachment figure and interactions with the attachment figure, as well as associated models of the self. For example, based on repeated experiences of the attachment figure's rejection of attempts to have his or her attachment needs met, the child forms an internal working model of the attachment figure as rejecting, of the self as unworthy, and expectations of rejection in interactions with the attachment figure.

As Bowlby (1973) notes, insofar as the formation of internal working models enables the child to better *predict* events he or she may confront, it serves an important adaptive function—even if, or perhaps especially if, the expected events are negative or threatening ones. For one thing, the internal working model provides stability, and for another thing, it permits the child to develop coping and defensive strategies, an issue that plays a major role in understanding different attachment patterns.

Bowlby (1973) maintained that the child's internal working models developed on the basis of "tolerably accurate" (p. 202) representations of repeated experiences with the caregiver. As he puts it, "the particular form that a person's working model takes is a fair reflection of the types of experiences he has had in his relationships with attachment figures" (Bowlby, p. 297). That is, they largely reflect actual events rather than fantasy. As one would expect, this claim became a major point of contention between Bowlby's attachment theory and the psychoanalytic strong emphasis on fantasy and psychic reality. Further, the notion that internal working models were largely based on actual events pointed to an emphasis on some form of environmental "failure"—usually in the form of the attachment figure's unavailability—in an etiological account of psychopathology. This was also at odds with the psychoanalytic emphasis on endogenous factors (e.g., intrapsychic conflict; the death instinct; the inherent antagonism between the id and the ego). These issues are discussed in later chapters. I turn now to what I referred to as important but secondary tenets.

INDIVIDUAL DIFFERENCES IN INTERNAL
WORKING MODELS AND ATTACHMENT PATTERNS

A highly generative and productive consequence of introducing the concept of internal working models lay in its implication of the existence of individual differences.[3] That is, if internal working models are the product of idiosyncratic interactions with the caregiver, it follows that there will be individual differences in internal working models as a function of differences in the nature of these interactions. Ainsworth et al.'s (1978) work in the development of the Strange Situation, their seminal observations and classification of differences in infants' behavioral patterns in the Strange Situations (referred to as "attachment style" or "attachment pattern"), and their linking these patterns to the infants' interactions with mother at home led to an explosion of research. As we see in the following chapter, a concern with individual differences in attachment patterns has virtually dominated attachment research.

There are many descriptions available of the Strange Situation and the attachment classifications derived from it (e.g., Ainsworth et al., 1978). Therefore, I only briefly summarize that information. The Strange Situation consists of a series of separations and reunions with the caregiver. It is mainly the infant's behavior during reunion that determines the infant's attachment classification. The infant who is classified as securely attached is someone who turns to the caregiver for comforting, is able to be comforted, and returns to play. Note that this infant is able to relate to caregiver as a safe haven and secure base. The avoidant–dismissive infant turns away from the caregiver upon reunion and/or ignores her and continues to play. The anxious–ambivalent infant is difficult to comfort and for a long period of time will continue to be distressed. Note that in both patterns of insecure attachment, the infant does not fully use caregiver as a safe haven or secure base. In addition to the above three categories, a fourth category, disorganized–disoriented has been identified that is characterized by bizarre behaviors such as freezing, twirling, walking backward, and lying flat under a table. Unlike the above organized categories, this classification suggests a breakdown in attachment organization rather than coherent coping (e.g., Main & Solomon, 1990). Disorganized–disoriented attachment has been associated with frightened–frightening caregiver behaviors,

---

[3]It should be noted that insofar as Bowlby attributed delinquency and other disturbances to the nature of the specific factors in the caregiver—child relationship, individual differences are already implied in his early work.

disruptive affective communication, and caregiver dissociation (Lyons-Ruth, Bronfman, & Parsons, 1999).

STABILITY OF ATTACHMENT PATTERNS

Bowlby (1973) proposed that once formed, attachment patterns and their underlying internal working models are relatively resistant to change. Thus, although the development of internal working models serves important adaptive functions, it also has maladaptive consequences, a main one of which is the power of internal working models to *assimilate* new experiences into preexisting schemas. One consequence of this tendency is a rigidity of preexisting sets of expectations and representations in relation to new significant figures. For example, if one approaches new relationships with an unyielding and rigid expectation of rejection and assimilates new experiences to that schema, it will be difficult to have a truly new experience that might serve to disconfirm the preexisting expectation of rejection. As we will see, this is an exceedingly important issue in the context of psychopathology and psychotherapy, particularly if one conceptualizes the former in terms of rigid and maladaptive schemas and the latter in terms of altering these rigid and maladaptive schemas.

An attempt to investigate the hypothesis that attachment patterns are relatively stable and resistant to change not only requires longitudinal studies, but also confronts one with issues of measurement. That is, in order to test whether attachment patterns are stable or change over time, one needs "ecologically valid" measures of attachment patterns at different points of time in the individual's life. I pursue this issue further in Chapter 4.

ATTACHMENT PATTERNS AND INTERNAL WORKING MODELS AS TRAIT-LIKE OR INTERACTIONAL

A question that arises is whether the attachment pattern is most meaningfully conceptualized as a stable trait-like personality characteristic or an interactional product that varies as a function of with whom one is interacting. Does one have a single internal working model that is stable across time and across different situations? Or does one have different internal working models that vary across time and with different individuals? The latter part of the question is meaningful only if one allows the possibility of multiple attachment figures who may be hierarchically arranged as well as being called upon as a function of a number of factors, including the nature of the challenge facing the child. For example, if the child's distress is due to illness, he or she may be more likely to call upon mother, whereas if the source of distress is physical, some children may be more likely to call upon father. Or, as another example, if one parent has been more available when the child explores, that parent may be more likely to function as a secure base for exploration. All this will depend on the history of the child's interactions with each parental figure and the internal working models resulting from those interactions.

As we see in subsequent chapters, much of the research in the literature treats attachment patterns as internal trait-like stable structures. This is partly based on the assumptions that (1) in the course of development we have one primary attachment figure, (2) the child's attachment pattern and underlying internal working models are based on interactions with that figure, (3) the internal working model and attachment pattern are relatively resistant to change, and (4) these early attachment patterns and internal working models are transferred to attachment figures later in life. Of course, these assumptions need to be examined further if one allows the possibilities of (1) more than one attachment figure and (2) a different set of experiences in interaction with this "additional" attachment figure.

ATTACHMENT AND DEVELOPMENT: ADULT ATTACHMENT

Bowlby (1979) writes that the importance of attachment bonds are present "from the cradle to the grave" (p. 129). However, the nature of one's attachment needs and the form in which they are expressed undoubtedly change in the course of development. As an obvious example, prior to the infant's ability to locomote, proximity to the caregiver will be achieved through the signal of crying. At a later stage, the infant can actively crawl or creep or walk to the caregiver. Although there is an attachment literature on attachment needs and their forms of expression over the course of development, most of that literature deals with adult attachment rather than the developmental trajectory from one to the other.

One obvious change in attachment behavior in the course of normal development is that one can achieve a psychological "proximity" to one's attachment figure through symbolic means rather than relying entirely on physical proximity. That is, an image, a memory, a photograph, a letter, or phone call can serve attachment functions that, for the young child, can only be served by physical proximity.

The "transitional object" that Winnicott (1953) has written about occupies a psychological space somewhere between requiring the physical presence of the caregiver in order to be comforted and being able to be comforted by a quasi-symbolic stand-in for the caregiver. Although the child needs to be in physical proximity to the transitional object in order to be comforted by it, its capacity to soothe in the first place is a symbolic capacity given to it by the child. The point here is that the capacity of the transitional object to comfort and soothe represents a way station on the road to an increasing autonomy from the need for actual physical proximity to the caregiver and an increasing internalization of safe haven and secure base functions.

In the course of development, peer relationships assume increasing importance in the life of the child, although for the young child, parents remain his or her attachment figure. However, as development proceeds toward adulthood, it is generally the case that one's romantic partner becomes one's primary attachment figure. That is, someone outside one's family of origin becomes one's primary love object or attachment figure.[4] Unlike infant–caregiver attachment, adult–adult relationships are more reciprocal (Weiss, 1982). One of the issues that has been given much research attention is the degree to which one's attachment pattern established early in life with one's caregiver is transferred to one's adult attachment figure. This issue is of special interest in a discussion of the relationship between attachment theory and psychoanalysis.

As noted, in order to shed light on such questions as stability of attachment patterns and transfer of early attachment patterns to current attachment figures, one needs to be able to measure adult attachment patterns. Two primary means of assessing adult attachment have emerged: the Adult Attachment Interview (AAI; Main & Goldwyn, 1998) and self-report questionnaires. The latter began with a relatively simple instrument (Hazan & Shaver, 1987) and has developed into a questionnaire, Experience in Close Relationships (ECR; Brennan, Clark, & Shaver, 1998), that taps the two dimensions of attachment anxiety and attachment avoidance.[5]

Corresponding to the categories in the Strange Situation, the AAI yields the following attachment classifications: secure–autonomous, avoidant–dismissive, and enmeshed–preoccupied. In addition, there is a

---

[4]Richard Bowlby (personal communication, 2008) conveyed to me what can be considered a one-question "test" to determine who one's attachment figure is: "Whom would you call if you were given very distressing news, such as being told that you have a serious, life-threatening illness?" It occurs to me that this works equally well if the question is: "Whom would you call if you received very good news such as winning the lottery?"

[5]Other instruments have been developed to measure adult attachment. I refer to the AAI and ECR because they are the most widely used instruments.

score for Unresolved for loss and trauma, which corresponds to the disorganized–disoriented classification in the Strange Situation.

These classifications are mainly determined by structural properties
of the individual's narrative. The property of the narrative that contributes
most heavily to the individual's attachment classification is the *coherence*
of the narrative. Thus, a narrative characterized by coherence between
general descriptions of parents (subjects are asked to provide a number of
adjectives that describe each parent) and instantiating concrete episodes
will be classified as secure–autonomous.

A narrative characterized by denigrating the importance of attachment
and incongruence between general descriptions of parents and concrete episodes or the inability to provide concrete instantiating episodes will be classified as avoidant–dismissive. Idealization of parents not supported or even
contradicted by concrete memories is a common feature of these narratives.

A narrative characterized by preoccupation with attachment issues, as
if the individual continues to be enmeshed in these issues, will be classified
as enmeshed–preoccupied. Evidence of such enmeshment and preoccupa-
tions includes a tendency toward incoherence between past and present
relationships, and a lack of distance, as if the individual remains preoccupied with the past.

The narratives that are classified as unresolved–disorganized, which
can also have one of the other major attachment categories as a secondary classification, are characterized by lapses in reasoning or discourse or
other anomalies when discussing experiences of loss or abuse. The inference underlying this classification is that the lack of resolution of loss or
abuse leads to cognitive lapses.

A general and important point to be noted with regard to the AAI
classifications is that they are intended to refer to the individual's state
of mind with respect to attachment (Main, 1991). Thus, as noted, a narrative classified as secure–autonomous is presumed to reflect a *coherent*
state of mind, whereas the other classifications are presumed, in one way
or another, to reflect an *incoherent* state of mind with respect to attachment.

The ECR yields the following attachment classifications: Low in
anxiety and low in avoidance defines secure attachment; high in anxiety
and low in avoidance defines anxious attachment; high in avoidance and
low in anxiety defines avoidant attachment; and high in avoidance and
high in anxiety defines fearful–avoidant attachment. Of special interest is
the capacity of the ECR to yield not only categories, but also *dimensions*
of degree of anxiety and degree of avoidance. And finally, it needs to be
noted that, whereas the AAI focuses on the individual's state of mind

with respect to his or her early attachment experiences (Main, 1991), the items on the ECR deal with the individual's *current* attachment relationship. Hence, it should not be surprising that, as we will see, the AAI and the ECR correlate only minimally with each other and predict different behaviors, suggesting that they measure different aspects of adult attachment (Crowell, Treboux, & Waters, 1999). (This issue will be pursued in Chapter 4.)

CHAPTER 3

Key Research Findings

In collaboration with Everett Waters

This chapter selectively covers representative research findings that deal with central ideas of attachment theory. The choice of research findings covered in this chapter was guided by my judgment of their importance and by their relevance to fundamental ideas of attachment theory. (For a comprehensive summary of attachment research, see the excellent *Handbook of Attachment*, edited by Cassidy & Shaver, 2008.)

THE ATTACHMENT SYSTEM AND PROXIMITY TO THE CAREGIVER

As Cassidy and Shaver (2008) point out, the most fundamental tenet of attachment theory is the positing of "a proclivity to seek proximity" to the caregiver which can be understood as "a behavioral adaptation in the same way that a fox's white coat on the tundra is an adaptation" (p. 5). The attachment behavioral system consists of various behaviors such as vocalizing and smiling that have the predictable outcome of achieving proximity to the caregiver. Bowlby (1969/1982) proposed that that these proximity-facilitating behaviors come together in the course of experience to constitute the attachment system. A fundamental biological function of that system is to enhance the infant's survival and, ultimately, reproductive fitness.

There is, of course, no set of definitive studies that one can point to that provide definitive evidence for this core tenet. Rather, it reflects an evolutionary framework in which behaviors are viewed in terms of their adaptation to environmental niches. However, the presence of proximity-seeking behavior at birth in other species, as well as in different human cultures, speak to their evolutionary origins.

AFFECT REGULATION AND PROXIMITY TO THE CAREGIVER

A basic assumption made by Bowlby is that relatively prolonged separation, threats of separation, and unavailability of the caregiver are anxiety-provoking to the infant, especially when he or she is already experiencing distress. A corollary of that assumption is that proximity to the caregiver is comforting (safe haven function) when the infant is distressed. In short, separation is affect dysregulating and proximity is affect regulating.

There is informal as well as systematic evidence in both animals and humans in support of the above propositions. With regard to the informal evidence, all one need do is observe the countless occasions of a child in distress being able to be comforted and soothed by his or her caregiver.

Working with rats, Hofer and his colleagues (e.g., Hofer, 2006; Polan & Hofer, 2008) have demonstrated that early in life the caregiver serves vital regulating functions and that the removal of these regulating functions through maternal separation causes dysregulation and distress in the infant. The mother regulates a wide range of the rat pup's physiological and behavioral systems through the provision of different kinds of stimulation (e.g., thermal, tactile, milk, olfactory). Each of these inputs regulates a particular system in the infant. For example, the provision of warmth regulates the infant's activity level; milk regulates heart rate; tactile stimulation regulates the infant's production of the growth hormone ornithine decarboxylase. With regard to the latter, in an attempt to develop an animal model of "psychosocial dwarfism," Schanberg and Kuhn (1980) have shown that the level of ornithine decarboxylase, which drops precipitously when the rat pup is separated from mother, can be brought back to a normal level if the infant rat is stroked for a set period every day with a wet brush that is similar to the texture of the mother's tongue.

EFFECTS OF EARLY SEPARATION, NEGLECT,
AND MALTREATMENT ON DEVELOPMENT

A basic assumption made by Bowlby is that separation, threats of separation, maltreatment, and so on at the hands of the caregiver are risk factors for later psychopathology and maladjustment (see Chapter 10). Indeed,
Bowlby's earliest interest and publications—the forerunners of attachment
theory—were concerned with the developmental consequences of these
early risk factors (see Chapter 1). Bowlby disputed the traditional psychoanalytic idea that because they had not yet developed object constancy
or the requisite ego functions, infants were not capable of mourning in
response to maternal separation or deprivation. Thus, research that demonstrates the negative consequences of early maternal separation, though
relevant to a number of theoretical developmental perspectives, is especially
important for attachment theory.

There is evidence demonstrating both the immediate and long-term
dysregulating effects of maternal separation. For example, Huot, Plotsky,
Lenox, and McNamara (2002) reported that daily neonatal maternal separation of 3-hour duration of rat pups at postnatal days 2–14 produced
increased basal levels of corticotropin releasing factor and enhanced adrenocorticotropic hormone and corticosterone in response to psychological
stressors. Furthermore, as adults, those rats "exhibited elevated indices of
anxiety, startle-induced pituitary–adrenal hyper-responsiveness" (p. 52)
and maze learning deficits. Similar effects were not reported when the
separation duration was only 15 minutes. In humans, there is evidence,
beginning with Ainsworth's (1967) classic work, that lack of caregiver
responsiveness is associated with insecure patterns of attachment.[1] There is
also evidence that insecure attachment patterns constitute risk factors for
psychopathology (see Chapter 10) and for physical health.

With regard to the latter, Maunder and Hunter (2001, 2008) have sur-
veyed the literature and have cited evidence supporting the hypothesis that
through a variety of different mechanisms, insecure attachment may contribute to poor physical health. For example, employing the Measurement
of Attachment Quality (MAQ), a 14-item self-report measure, Gallo and
Matthews (2006) found that adolescents high in attachment anxiety show
high diastolic and systolic blood pressure when interacting with friends
and that adolescents high in avoidance show higher diastolic blood pressure in conflictual interactions compared to securely attached individuals.

---

[1] As we will see, although caregiver's sensitive responsiveness is correlated with the infant's attachment status, the relationship is not as robust as attachment theory would predict.

Insecurely attached individuals show elevated cortisol response to relationship conflict (Powers, Pietromonaco, Gunlicks, & Sayer, 2006). Although individuals with fearful avoidant attachment report the highest levels of symptoms, they show the lowest level of health care utilization, thus running the risk of failing to treat possible illness.

A similar dynamic seems to be at work with avoidantly attached diabetic patients. Employing the Relationship Scale Questionnaire, a 30-item self-report measure, Ciechanowski, Katon, and Hirsch (2002) reported that 62% of diabetic patients with dismissing attachment had a mean glycosylated hemoglobin (HbAlc) of 8 or greater, compared with 34% of securely attached diabetic patients. Since HbAlc is the primary measure of long-term diabetic control, these findings suggest that the dismissing patients were not adequately monitoring diet and medication. As a final example of the relationship between attachment pattern and physical health, Sloan, Maunder, Hunter, and Moldofsky (2007) found that insecure attachment was associated with elevated levels of alpha wave activity in sleep which, in turn, is associated with nonrestorative sleep.

THE ATTACHMENT FIGURE AS A SECURE BASE FOR THE CHILD'S EXPLORATORY ACTIVITY

The informal evidence for the proposition that the attachment figure serves as a secure base for the infant's and children exploratory activity is overwhelming. Observing the immediate cessation of play and exploration and their replacement by distress when a toddler playing at a sandbox turns and does not see mother is a familiar example of such evidence. However, a wealth of more systematic evidence can be presented in both animals and humans attesting to the secure base function of the caregiver.

With regard to animal studies, recall the replacement of distress and fear by exploratory activity in Harlow's (1958) monkeys (cited in Chapter 2) when confronted with a toy "monster" when the terry cloth surrogate mother was present versus absent; and Rajecki et al.'s (1978) finding that in every species studied—dogs, chicks, monkeys, and children—exploratory activity increases when the attachment figure is present.

There are also a number of studies (cited in Chapter 2) with children on the relationship between the availability of the attachment figure and exploratory activity. As we have seen in one study, the mere presence of a photograph of mother increased the child's exploratory activity (Passman & Erck, 1977; Passman & Longeway, 1982). In another study, over and above physical availability, mother's emotional availability (i.e., reading a newspaper vs. being fully available) increased exploratory activity (Sorce & Emde, 1981).

There is also evidence on the relationship between the availability of a secure base and not only the range, but also the quality of exploratory activity—that is, whether the exploratory activity is relatively defensive or nondefensive, comfortable or accompanied by anxiety. For example, Sroufe and Waters (1977) reported that the exploratory activity of avoidant infants—who presumably do not adequately experience their caregiver as a secure base—is accompanied by increased heart rate, suggesting that such activity is defensive and relatively anxiety-laden rather than experienced as comfortable and gratifying.

INDIVIDUAL DIFFERENCES IN ATTACHMENT PATTERNS AND INTERNAL WORKING MODELS AS A FUNCTION OF INTERACTIONS WITH THE CAREGIVER

As noted in Chapter 2, Bowlby proposed that, based on repeated interactions, the child develops an internal working model of what to expect from the caregiver (which also includes self-representations and representations of the attachment figure based on these interactions). Hence, different interactions will generate different internal working models and correspondingly different attachment patterns.

Although the mere existence of individual differences in attachment patterns is not a core proposition of attachment theory, by far the greatest number of attachment studies have dealt with such individual differences. In order for individual differences in attachment patterns to be directly relevant to the core propositions of attachment theory, one would need to show that they are lawfully related to relevant variations in caregiver behavior. However, although the caregiver's behavior is, indeed, correlated with the infant's attachment status, with the exception of the relationship between caregiver behavior and disorganized attachment, the relationship between the two has not been a robust one. That is, mother's sensitive responsiveness accounts for less of the variance in predicting infant's attachment status (e.g., Raval et al., 2001) than one would expect based on the logic of attachment theory. This has been referred to as the "transmission gap."

There are a number of ways of understanding the "transmission gap." One plausible explanation is that in contrast to Ainsworth's careful assessment of mother's behavior, more recent assessments in many studies tend to be "quick and dirty" (Everett Waters, personal communication, 2007). It may be that measures based on careful, lengthy, and detailed assessments of mother's behavior would show a stronger relationship to the child's attachment status. Thus, the lack of a robust relationship might largely be a measurement problem. That is, as De Wolff and van IJzendoorn (1997) put it, "the much weaker associations can ... be attributed to methodological weaknesses of the replication studies" (p. 572), including observations based on a single home visit or brief laboratory assessments. Supporting this argument is the fact that studies that are closer in design to the original Ainsworth study tend to yield a stronger association between maternal sensitivity and child attachment status (e.g., Isabella, 1993; Pederson et al., 1990).

In order to bring "some degree of order to a large and inconsistent body of findings" (p. 572), De Wolff and van IJzendoorn (1997) carried out a highly sophisticated meta-analysis involving 66 studies and 4,176 mother–infant pairs that addressed a number of hypotheses regarding the relationship between maternal behavior and infant attachment. Using Cohen's (1988) criteria, a medium effect size was found between maternal sensitivity and security of attachment, which was somewhat larger when the studies used the original Ainsworth, Bell, and Stayton (1974) sensitivity scale. The authors conclude that "after more than 25 years of research, Bowlby's (1969/1982) important question about the role of sensitivity in the development of infant attachment can therefore be answered in the affirmative" (p. 584). They also conclude that although the meta-analysis found that maternal sensitivity is an important factor in infant attachment security, the relationship between the two was found to be weaker than the relationship found in the original Ainsworth et al. (1978) study.

An extremely important finding of the meta-analysis is that maternal behaviors other than sensitivity—for example, mutuality, synchrony, stimulation, positive attitude, and emotional support—showed a relationship to attachment security similar to sensitivity. As the authors note, "sensitivity has lost its privileged position as the only important causal factor" (p. 585) and needs to give way to a "multidimensional approach to parental antecedents" (p. 585). Other findings are also worth noting. For example, socioeconomic status, age of infant, interval between sensitivity and attachment assessments, all appear to moderate the relationship between sensitivity and attachment. As the authors note, other maternal behaviors that have not been adequately studied, such as discipline and management, may also be significantly linked to infant attachment. And finally, as the role of socioeconomic status suggests, contextual factors may strongly influence and even override the effects of maternal sensitivity.

An additional possible reason for only a modest relationship between maternal sensitivity and infant attachment has emerged from an exciting new area of research on molecular genetics and attachment. Belsky and his colleagues have speculated that there is variation in infants' susceptibility to rearing influence (Belsky, 1997a, 1997b, 2005; Belsky, Bakermans-Kranenburg, & van IJzendoorn, 2007; Belsky, Hsieh, & Crnic, 1998). Such variation would attenuate the overall relationship between maternal behaviors, including sensitivity, and infant attachment status. Future studies should focus on interaction as well as main effects (see Chapter 11).

In support of Belsky's hypothesis, Bakermans-Kranenberg et al. (2008) have provided fascinating evidence suggesting that the relationship between parental behavior and infant and child attachment status is moderated by the latter's genetically based differential susceptibility to environmental influence. For example, they have presented evidence that the presence of the dopamine D4 receptor (DRD4) 7-repeat polymorphism in children is associated with an increased risk of an 18.8-fold magnitude for disorganized attachment, but only when combined with environmental risk, including maternal anomalous behavior (see also van IJzendoorn & Bakermans-Kranenberg, 2006). However, there is also suggestive evidence that children with the DRD4 7-repeat allele fare *better* when exposed to a positive child-rearing environment (Bakermans-Kranenberg, van IJzendoorn, Mesman, Alink, & Jutter, 2008). These findings support Belsky (2005) and Belsky et al.'s (2007) hypothesis that some children are differentially susceptible to *both* negative *and* positive parental behaviors.

It might also be the case that at least some of the mother's behaviors that would be more robustly predictive of infant's attachment status are too subtle to be captured by relatively gross measures. This possibility is suggested by the work of Beebe and her colleagues (2010), who have been able to predict the infant's attachment status at 1 year of age based on observing filmed micro interactions between infant and mother during the first 4 months of the infant's life. They found that self-contingency, that is, the degree of stability versus lability over time in a variety of modalities (e.g., gaze, touch, facial expression), as well as the infant contingent coordination with mother at 4 months of age, was predictive of the infant's attachment status at 1 year of age. They note that "contrary to dominant theories in the literature on face-to-face interaction, measures of maternal contingent coordination with infant yielded the fewest associations with 12-month attachment" (p. 6). "Thus, the ways that infants regulated their own behaviors, and coordinated their behavior with mothers, and the ways that mothers regulated their own behaviors, gave two to three times more information about future 12-month infant attachment status than the ways that mothers coordinated their behavior with the infant's prior behavior"

(p. 113). The infant and mother behaviors and interactions noted by Beebe et al. would be difficult to observe through ordinary means.

Raval et al. (2001) wanted to determine whether they could explain or reduce the "transmission gap" by assessing maternal sensitivity specifically in the context of attachment-relevant behaviors (e.g., protective behavior) and in situations in which the mother's attention was divided—a situation that often characterizes mother's state. With regard to the latter, previous work had shown that the relationship between maternal sensitivity and infant attachment was stronger when mothers had to divide their attention than when mothers were focused on their infant.

Mother–infant interaction during a divided attention task was video-taped when infant was 6 months of age. The results showed that while mother's responsiveness to *clear* infant signals at 6 months was not significantly related to infant's attachment status at 1 year, responsiveness to *possible* signals showed a significant relationship to infant attachment. Despite this significant relationship and the attempt to "improve" operational definitions of maternal responsiveness, the study essentially replicated van IJzendoorn's (1995) meta-analysis finding that maternal responsiveness contributes relatively modestly to infant attachment status. Raval et al. (2001) conclude that there is a serious possibility that some part of the transmission is genetic.

And, indeed, there is some evidence suggesting a genetic component to attachment status (e.g., Finkel, Wille, & Matheny, 1998; van IJzendoorn et al., 2000)—although there is also contrary evidence (see Roisman & Fraley, 2006, however, for a discussion of the limits of genetic influence in accounting for variations in infant–caregiver relationships). Raval et al. (2001) also note that maternal responsiveness is only one aspect of infant–mother interactions and suggest that other aspects of the interaction (e.g., openness of communication) may influence infant attachment status. We have seen examples of some of these other aspects in the Beebe et al. (2010) study. And finally, they stress the need to explore various domains of the mother's behavior as well as the infant's general social and psychological context in understanding the infant's attachment status.

DISORGANIZED ATTACHMENT AND CAREGIVER BEHAVIOR

Although measures of mother's sensitive responsiveness are not as robust in predicting secure and insecure attachment classifications in the Strange Situation as one would expect based on attachment theory, certain of the mother's behaviors—for example, frightened–frightening behavior, disrupted affective communication, and abusive and neglectful behavior—are more strongly predictive of the infant's *disorganized* attachment (Lyons-Ruth, Bronfman, & Parsons, 1999; Main & Hesse, 1995).

As noted in Chapter 2, in addition to the three attachment patterns observed by Ainsworth, all of which can be understood as *organized* strategies and adaptations to the caregiver's behavior, a *disorganized, disoriented* form of attachment has been identified that can coexist with other attachment patterns (Main & Solomon, 1990). Infant behaviors during the reunion phase of the Strange Situation that are bizarre and seem devoid of any coherent strategy designed to have one's attachment needs met (e.g., freezing; twirling; trance-like expression; crawling under the table) are the primary criteria for the disorganized attachment designation.

Main and Hesse (1995) have proposed that disorganized attachment is likely to be associated with caregiver's frightened–frightening behavior. Their reasoning was essentially that when the caregiver herself or himself is a source of distress (through being frightened and therefore not available or through emitting frightening behavior), there is an activation of two incompatible systems (fear and attachment), with the result that no coherent strategy is available to the infant. In an attempt to identify caregiver behaviors that are associated with infant disorganization, Hesse and Main (2006) developed six scales to identify varieties of such behavior: (1) Threatening, (2) Frightened, (3) Dissociative, (4) Timid or deferential, (5) Spousal or romantic, and (6) Disorganized.

In addition to frightening–frightened behavior, investigators have found other maternal behaviors that are associated with infant attachment disorganization. Lyons-Ruth and her colleagues (e.g., Lyons-Ruth et al., 1999) developed a coding system to measure disrupted forms of communication between infant and caregiver. It is called the Atypical Maternal Behavior Instrument for Assessment and Classification (AMBIANCE) and includes scales of Negative-intrusive behavior, Role confusion, Affective communication errors, and Disorientation. Lyons-Ruth, Connell, Grunebaum, and Botein (1990) found that level of affective communicative errors in the Strange Situation significantly predicted infant attachment disorganization. This finding has been replicated by a number of investigators (e.g., Gervai et al., 2007; Grienenberger, Kelly, & Slade, 2005). In addition, a meta-analysis by Madigan, Moran, Schuengel, Pederson, and Otten (2007) showed a significant relationship between disrupted communication and infant attachment disorganization ($r = .35$, $N = 384$).[2]

---

[2]However, it is important to note that a relatively high level of disrupted communication was also found in a low-risk sample of secure infants (Goldberg, Benoit, Blokland, & Madigan, 2003). This suggests that the relationship between disrupted communication and disorganization is not a simple one and is likely to include other factors.

Neglect and generally terrible conditions are also associated with disorganized attachment. Zeanah, Smyke, Koga, Carlson, and the Bucharest Group (2005) reported that 78% of 12–31-month-old institutionalized infants in Romania showed disorganized attachment. Carlson, Cicchetti, Barnett, and Braunwald (1989) reported that 82% of maltreated children were disorganized compared to 18% of a low-income control group. And Cicchetti and Curtis (2006) reported that 90% of maltreated children were disorganized compared to 43% for a low-income control group (which is an exceptionally high percentage).

In a study with pregnant women whose immediately prior pregnancy ended in stillbirth, Hughes, Turton, Hopper, McCauley, and Fonagy (2001) found a significant association between unresolved status on the AAI and infant disorganization. Also, infant disorganization was independently predicted by mother having seen her stillborn child in her past pregnancy or having elective termination of her earlier pregnancy. One can speculate that the mother's unresolved traumatic experience in a prior pregnancy may have led to anomalous behavior (e.g., being frightened) in relation to her infant. Consistent with this interpretation, Manassis, Bradley, Goldberg, Hood, and Swinson (1994) found that 65% of children of anxiety-disordered mothers showed disorganized attachment. Most of these mothers were unresolved in relation to loss or trauma on the AAI. (Also, see Abrams, Rifkin, & Hesse, 2006; Jacobvitz, Leon, & Hazen, 2006; Lyons-Ruth et al., 1999.)[3]

CAREGIVER AAI CLASSIFICATION
AND INFANT'S STRANGE SITUATION CLASSIFICATION

One of the puzzling findings that emerge from research in this area is that the caregiver's categorization on the AAI is more strongly related to the infant's attachment status than to direct measures of her behavior. If as Main (1991) notes, the AAI measures the caregiver's "state of mind with respect to attachment," one would have to conclude that mother's state of mind is more strongly related to her infant's attachment status than her behavior. But this conclusion appears to make little sense. Unless the caregiver's state of mind is reflected in her behavior toward her child in some way, how could it influence the child? One's states of mind alone do not influence another.

---

[3]In at least one study, Schuengel, Bakermans-Kranenburg, & van IJzendoorn (1999) found only a marginal relationship between frightening/frightened maternal behavior and infant disorganization.

As noted above, one possible explanation for this state of affairs is that mother's classification on the AAI is associated with subtle behaviors that may not be captured by the usual assessments. Whether this is so awaits further research. However, some indirect evidence tends to support this hypothesis. Fonagy et al. (1995) have shown that most of the variance on the AAI is accounted for by individual differences in reflective functioning. Furthermore, Fonagy et al. have also reported that mother's capacity for reflective functioning on the AAI is strongly associated with infant's attachment status, particularly with high-risk mothers (i.e., single mothers, low socioeconomic status, etc.). That is to say, mother's capacity to reflect on her mental states with regard to her own early attachment experiences is predictive of her infant's attachment status. This suggests that because she remembers or, more accurately, reflects rather than repeats, she is better able to respond to her infant contingently rather than repeat a rigid pattern originating in her own attachment experience. What is needed, however, to support this hypotheses is research relating maternal reflective functioning and careful assessments of mother's behaviors, including subtle behaviors, toward her infant.[4]

RELATIONSHIP BETWEEN INFANT ATTACHMENT PATTERNS AND COGNITIVE AND SOCIAL FUNCTIONING

According to attachment theory, secure attachment is likely to be associated with a more positive developmental trajectory in a number of areas than insecure attachment. Further, although attachment theorists caution that insecure attachment patterns do not constitute psychopathology, they are nevertheless seen as risk factors, whereas secure attachment is seen as a protective factor. There is also evidence that security of attachment is associated with greater cognitive and social competence.

With regard to the former, early attachment status predicts cognitive competence in middle childhood (Aviezer, Sagi, Resnick, & Gini, 2002). Analyzing data from the National Institute of Child Health and Human Development Study of Early Child Care, Belsky and Fearon (2002) found that security of attachment at 15 months was predictive of a broad range of cognitive capacities at 36 months.

As for social competence, Fonagy (1997) has shown that children

---

[4]To be noted here is the relevance of the psychoanalytic emphasis on awareness and enhancing the observing function of the ego as a means of altering maladaptive patterns acquired early in life. As we see in Chapter 11, this convergence between attachment and psychoanalytic theories underlies the rationale for virtually all infant–mother intervention programs.

securely attached in infancy show better understanding of others' affective states at age 5 than children who were insecurely attached in infancy. There is evidence that insecurely attached children are more dependent and seek more attention from teachers and camp counselors. This remains true at age 15. Also, preschool children with an avoidant history are more likely to victimize their play partner (Troy & Sroufe, 1987). Jacobson and Wille (1986) reported that although insecurely attached toddlers make as many social overtures as securely attached toddlers, they are chosen significantly less frequently as a playmate, which is to say that they are rejected significantly more frequently. That insecurely attached children "pull for" different responses, not only from peers but also from adults, is attested to by finding that both teachers and camp counselors respond differently to securely and insecurely attached children.

If one is to break into this vicious circle, one needs to identify the factors that account for the more frequent rejection of the insecure toddler found in the Jacobson and Wille (1986) study. The other toddlers who reject the insecure toddler's social overtures must be responding to some behavioral cues. What are they? This study cries out for follow-up research aimed at identifying these cues. Similarly follow-up is needed for the earlier reported finding that insecurely attached children pull for responses from teachers and camp counselors that are different from securely attached children.[5]

These findings suggest the potential self-fulfilling nature of the insecurely attached child's interactions with peers and adults. That is, the internal working model of the insecurely attached child is assumed to include expectations of rejection, representations of significant figures as rejecting, and representations of self as unworthy. The child is then likely to behave in precisely the way that will lead to rejection and reinforce his or her preexisting internal working model. This is a powerful dynamic that would serve to maintain and perpetuate an early internal working model of one's self as unworthy and of others as rejecting.

DISORGANIZED ATTACHMENT
AND COGNITIVE AND SOCIAL FUNCTIONING

The above findings suggest that whereas most infants may be able to "handle" a wide range of caregiver behaviors through organized attachment

---

[5] A similar dynamic is also implicit in the concept of transference and is a central consideration in the psychoanalytic or psychodynamic conception of treatment. The patient comes to treatment with a transference pattern, that is, with a set of expectations and representations, that, as Strupp and Binder (1984) point out, "pull for" certain responses from the therapist.

strategies, behaviors outside the range of an "average expectable environment" (Hartmann, 1958)—for example, abuse and maltreatment—disrupt attachment organization.

A number of studies have investigated the relationship between early disorganization and later development. Some typical correlates of early attachment disorganization include: controlling behavior that is either controlling or punitive at age 6 (Main & Cassidy, 1988; Wartner, Grossmann, Fremmer-Bombik, & Suess, 1994); poorer performance on syllogistic reasoning at ages 9–17 (Jacobsen, Edelstein, & Hofmann, 1994); poor school performance at ages 5–7 and greater externalizing and internalizing problems (Moss & Rousseau, 1998; Moss, St-Laurent, & Parent, 1999); less competence in quality of play with peers and less ability to resolve conflicts, although no less competence than avoidant children (Warner et al., 1994); higher levels of anger (Kochanska, 2001); more dissociative behavior in high school (Carlson, 1998; Ogawa, Sroufe, Weinfield, Carlson, & Egeland, 1997); and greater susceptibility to experiencing trauma later in life (Ogawa et al., 1997).

STABILITY OF ATTACHMENT PATTERNS

Although working models can change as a function of new experiences (Bowlby, 1973), an assumption of attachment theory is that attachment patterns and their underlying working models established early in life are relatively resistant to change, that is, tend to remain relatively stable from infancy to adulthood. What is the evidence for the stability hypothesis?

The path that has been taken in the relatively few long-term longitudinal studies carried out is to compare the infant's attachment pattern in the Strange Situation with the individual's attachment classification on the AAI in adulthood. The results have been mixed. Sroufe, Egeland, Carlson, and Collins (2005a) found no significant relationship between attachment classification at 12 months in the Strange Situation and AAI classification at age 19. However, they did find modest stability between infant classifications at 18 months and AAI at age 26. However, the stability was entirely due to the relationship between secure at 18 months and secure–autonomous at 26 years of age. Sroufe et al. (2005) suggest that these findings may be due to the greater stability of attachment at 18 months.

Waters, Merrick, Treboux, Crowell, and Albersheim (2000) administered the AAI to a group of 20-year-olds after they had been given the Strange Situation at 12 and 18 months of age. They found that 70% of the participants received the same attachment classifications using the

secure–insecure dimension; and that 64% were assigned the same classification in infancy and adulthood using the three attachment classifications
of secure, insecure–avoidant, and insecure–resistant. Change in attachment
classification from infancy to adulthood was significantly related to reports
of negative life events such as loss, parental divorce, and physical and sexual abuse. Most of the changes were from secure to insecure as a function
of these negative life events. The authors conclude that the findings support
Bowlby's hypothesis that attachment patterns are relatively stable, but are
open to change in the light of real-life experiences. It is important to keep
in mind that the Waters et al. (2000) sample was a stable middle-class one,
whereas the Sroufe et al. (2005a) sample was a high-risk one.

Perhaps more important than looking for evidence of stability—or
instability—of attachment patterns is an understanding of the factors that
make for stability or instability, or what Sroufe et al. (2005a) refer to as
"lawful discontinuity." As noted, an important factor that contributes to
stability of attachment patterns over time is the stability of the individual's
caregiving environment. When the environment is unstable and marked by
changes such as divorce and loss, attachment patterns tend to change (e.g.,
Lewis, Feiring, & Rosenthal, 2000).

This suggests that when stability of attachment patterns is found the
kinds of early experiences and interactions associated with the infant's
attachment status are likely repeated at different stages of development.
Thus, a caregiver who is sensitively responsive when the infant is 12 or 18
months of age is more likely to be sensitively responsive in an age-appro-
priate way when the child is 3 or 4 or 5. Conversely, a caregiver who is not
sensitively responsive when the infant is 12 or 18 months of age is more
likely to show a similar pattern of behavior when the child is older.

Thus, when stability is found, it is not necessarily that some structure
formed in infancy (e.g., attachment pattern or internal working model) that
remains relatively unchanged during the course of development untouched
by later experiences influences later development. Rather, it is likely that
later experiences serve either to maintain or change these early structures.
For example, with regard to the former, let us say that in response to
repeated rejection at the hands of his or her caregiver, the infant develops
an avoidant–dismissive attachment pattern and an internal working model
that includes expectations of rejection from the attachment figure. And let
us also say—forgetting for the moment measurement issues—that as an
adult the individual is also avoidant–dismissive. One way of accounting
for such stability is that, given the resistance to change, the individual's
internal working model established early in life has remained static and
unchanged—the attachment theory counterpart to Freud's (1915/1963,

p. 187) "timelessness" of the unconscious and his assumption that adult neurosis is largely a reemergence of an "infantile neurosis."

This way of looking at things, however, is likely to be inaccurate and not representative of the nature of developmental processes. What is rather likely to be the case is that when there is stability between early and adult internal working models, it is, in large part at least, due to a variety of maintaining factors. The stability of the environment is a maintaining factor. There are likely to be other factors. For example, in discussing the Jacobson and Wille (1986) finding that insecure toddlers are more frequently rejected as playmates, I noted that these toddlers undoubtedly emit cues that elicit rejection responses from other children that serve to reinforce the rejected child's internal working model.[6] In general eliciting behaviors from others that serve to reinforce existing working models may be a powerful maintaining factor.

Later in life, choice of a mate, or what is referred to in the psychoanalytic context as object choice, is also likely to be a factor that makes for stability of attachment pattern. Evidence that parental figures serve as a template for object choice (Freud, 1931/1961, p. 228) would provide support for the hypothesis that object choice contributes to stability of attachment patterns (see Fraley & Marks, 2010). The phenomenon of positive assortative mating—that is, the tendency to choose a mate similar to oneself and one's family (Bereczkei, Gyuris, Koves, & Bernaths, 2002; Zajonc, Adelmann, Murphy, & Niedenthal, 1987) can also be seen as contributing to stability of attachment patterns.

The longitudinal studies that have investigated the issue of the stability of attachment patterns generally focus on the trajectory from infancy to adulthood. Indeed, in a 2005 edited book on the major longitudinal studies, the title of which is *Attachment from Infancy to Adulthood*, all the studies cover the time period from infancy to adulthood (Grossmann, Grossmann, & Waters, 2005). However, in one of the few studies of its kind, Klohnen and Bera (1998) carried out a longitudinal study at different periods of adulthood from ages 21 to 52 in a group of 142 women. They assessed the attachment pattern through use of the relatively simple Hazan and Shaver (1987) questionnaire, which asks respondents to endorse one of three paragraphs presumably describing secure, avoidant, and preoccupied

---

[6]Bowlby (1988, pp. 135–136) contrasts a linear developmental theory that is analogous to a simple railway track going from A to endpoint N with a model of multiple tracks in which one goes from the starting point A to switching points B or C, each of which goes off in a different direction. Thus, referencing the Jacobson and Wille study, one can speculate that a toddler who has few playmates will develop fewer social skills, which, in turn, will facilitate developmental pathway A rather than developmental pathway B (see Rutter, Quinton, & Hill, 1990).

attachment patterns (the ECR was not available when the data were collected). In addition, the following assessments were also included: At age 21, based on observations of the women in formal and informal situations as part of the Mills Longitudinal Study, observers described the women with the California Adult Q-Set (CAQ; Block, 1978). At age 43, judges made ratings based on "extensive archival files" (p. 212). Other data were obtained, including self-descriptions on the Adjective Check List (ACL; Gough & Heilbrun, 1983), which the authors view as reflecting internal working models, information about childhood, and relationship outcomes.

The significant relationships between the Hazan and Shaver (1987) measure of attachment patterns and other variables were quite remarkable given the simplicity of the measurement of attachment patterns. Of the women who were avoidantly attached at age 52, 50% were not married compared to 18% of securely attached women (there were too few women who were preoccupied to include in the analysis). Of those who did marry, 50% of the avoidant women were divorced, compared to 24% of the secure women. At age 43, the average length of the longest relationship of avoidant women was two-thirds as long as that of securely attached women. Finally, early loss of parent, fewer siblings, and growing up in cities significantly predicted avoidant attachment.

Since attachment pattern was measured only at age 52, one can only infer stability based on other measures. Thus, the avoidantly attached women at age 52 showed higher distrust, greater emotional distance, and greater self-reliance over a 25-year period (i.e., from age 27 to age 52). Klohnen and Bera (1998) conclude that despite the fact that "attachment classifications were obtained only at a single point in time ... nonetheless, our findings from three different data sources (life data, observer descriptions, and self-reports) converged to provide robust evidence for the continuity of the behavioral and experiential patterns associated with attachment style" (p. 220).

We know that infants and children have relatively little control over the environments in which they find themselves. However, this is much less the case in adulthood. The women in the Klohnen and Bera (1998) study had a role in *selecting their environment*. Thus, the women who were avoidantly attached at age 52 already at age 21 "tended to differ in their relationship goals and values, expressing less interest in marriage and having a family" (p. 219). In short, a factor that is likely to influence and maintain stability of attachment patterns in adulthood is our tendency to place ourselves in environments that are congruent with our attachment pattern.

Although Bowlby argues that internal working models are relatively resistant to change—that is why I have devoted a good deal of space to the question of stability of attachment patterns—an equally important issue is an understanding of what Sroufe et al. (2005a) refer to as "lawful discontinuity" when there is an instability of attachment patterns. It seems to me that the stability of attachment patterns as a core tenet of attachment theory has been overemphasized. More important to the development of attachment theory is an adequate explanatory account of the factors involved in lawful continuity and lawful discontinuity. A more sophisticated and probably more realistic approach to the question of stability would lie in conditional hypotheses positing that attachment patterns will remain relatively stable under such and such conditions and will change in a particular direction under another specified set of conditions (see Sroufe et al.).

DO EARLY ATTACHMENT PATTERNS "TRANSFER" TO ADULT RELATIONSHIPS?

A variation or perhaps implication of the stability of attachment pattern issue is the assumption that the individual's attachment pattern and underlying working model established in relation to early caregiver tend to be "transferred" to current attachment figure. For example, one's early expectation of rejection associated with an avoidant attachment pattern is assumed to be operative in one's current attachment relationship.[7]

On this view the individual's preset early expectations and representations constitute the main determinants of his or her experience of the current attachment figure rather than the latter's actual behavior and characteristics. How would one go about investigating whether and to what degree attachment patterns established early in life with one's caregivers are "transferred" to one's current attachment figure. Thinking in terms of measurement issues, the AAI will not do insofar as it addresses relationships with parents, not current partners.

From a logical point of view, a more direct route to investigating the question would be a comparison of early attachment pattern yielded by the Strange Situation and attachment pattern in relation to current attachment figure. But the most frequently used instruments that measure attachment pattern in relation to current attachment figure are self-report measures,

---

[7]Note that implicit in this assumption is a trait-like conception of attachment patterns. That is, one's early attachment pattern (i.e., one's early expectations regarding the availability of one's attachment figure plus one's coping strategy) is assumed to be operative in relation to one's current attachment figure relatively independently of who that attachment figure is and independently of his or her actual availability.

such as the ECR. I know of no studies that have taken that route. Aside from the very different research traditions of the Strange Situation and the AAI, on the one hand, and self-report questionnaires such as the ECR, on the other, there are perhaps good reasons for the failure of such a study to be carried out. Longitudinal studies involving the Strange Situation and self-report questionnaire measures of attachment are not likely to be especially fruitful.

We know (1) that a relatively robust relationship is generally found between the Strange Situation and AAI classifications; and (2) that there is a very low correlation between AAI and self-report measures of attachment. Roisman et al.'s (2007) meta-analysis involving 900 subjects of all studies that included both the AAI and a self-report measure of attachment found a correlation of .09 between the two measures. Furthermore, each measure predicted different aspects of adult attachment functioning (see Waters, Crowell, Elliot, Corcoran, & Treboux, 2002). Despite this low correlation between them, it is statistically possible for each measure to correlate significantly with the Strange Situation. However, it is unlikely that one would find a significant relationship between the Strange Situation and a self-report measure.

There is some evidence of consistency between adult attachment pattern as measured by self-report and retrospective accounts of parent–child relationships (Collins & Read, 1990; Feeney & Noller, 1990; Hazan & Shaver, 1987). However, the significance of these findings is limited by the retrospective nature of the reports of parent–child relationships as well as the possible influence of current relationships on these reports.

In one study, employing interview methods to assess working models of *both* current relationships with parents and romantic partners, some degree of similarity was found (Owens, Crowell, Pan, & Treboux, 1995). Similarly employing interview methods, Furman, Simon, and Shaffer (2002) investigated the relationship among AAI, Romantic Relationship Interview, and Friendship Interview in a group of adolescents. A perhaps surprising finding was a stronger relationship between working models of parents and friends than between parents and romantic partner. Only preoccupied ratings for relationships with parents and romantic partner robustly related to each other. Also, there was a relatively high degree of concordance between working models of friends and romantic partner. In interpreting these findings one must keep in mind that (1) one's romantic partner in an adolescent relationship is not likely to serve as an attachment figure—for one thing, the relationship is not of sufficient longevity; (2) during the transitional stage that constitutes adolescence, one's close friendships are likely to be of longer duration than one's romantic relationships; and (3) accordingly, and in certain respects, one's close friends may be more likely to serve attachment functions than one's romantic partner.

There is some evidence that attachment classification on the AAI and secure base behaviors (e.g., seeking and providing support) in adult couple's interaction are correlated (e.g., Crowell et al., 2002; Wampler, Riggs, & Kimball, 2004). These findings are especially important because they link classification on the AAI narrative to actual "real-life" behavior that plays a central role in attachment theory. As a final example of consistency between working model of attachment to parents and current relationships, Crowell et al. found a substantial correlation ($r = .51$) between security scores obtained from the AAI and Current Relationship Interview (CRI).

ACTUAL EVENTS VERSUS FANTASY

Although it is generally thought of as a background assumption, one can view as a core tenet of attachment theory the claim that actual events in the early life of the child have a far greater influence on development than endogenously generated fantasies. It would be extremely difficult to test this hypothesis directly in a specific study. Rather, one can reasonably evaluate this claim by appealing to cumulative evidence and to what we know about infant capacities and infant development. And when one does this, the verdict is quite clear. Although it is difficult to prove a negative, no evidence at all exists that young infants are capable of the kinds of complex and florid fantasies attributed to them by Klein, or that, as Isaacs (1943/2003) maintained, reality is constructed out of fantasy. Rather, what we do know about infants strongly supports Stern's (1985) conclusion that the infant is "unapproachable by psychodynamic considerations for an initial period, resulting in a non-psychodynamic beginning of life" (p. 255).

Because much of the infant's experience is opaque, it is fertile ground for the projection of all sorts of adult fantasies. Much of the evidence indicates that generally speaking, the actual state of affairs is opposite to the standard psychoanalytic view that fantasy and wish-fulfillment characterize the psychic life of the infant and young child and that realistic thinking becomes increasingly evident as the child matures. From the very beginning the infant is reality oriented at its level of cognitive organization, although the manner and form of encoding information from the environment may not be the same as the adult's or the older child's. For example, Spelke (1990) has shown that as early as 3 months of age, infants are able to infer the continuous existence of objects moving out of view. As Gergely (1992) observes, much of the infant research suggests that young infants perceive and order the world not so much in terms of concrete features of objects, but rather in terms of more abstract amodal properties and cross-modal invariances such as place, path of movement, boundary, intensity, and rhythm. As Gergely also points out, these findings do not support the Kleinian view of the infant as possessing a repertoire of inborn object images such as breasts and penises. It is very likely that the young infant simply does not order experience this way.

The above kind of evidence strongly suggests that early in life, the infant is busy acquiring procedural knowledge of the way the world, including the interpersonal world, works. As Bowlby (1973), Stern (1985), and Beebe and Lachmann (1994), using terms such as "internal working model," "representations of interactions generalized" (RIGs), and "interactional structures" suggest, the infant is busy abstracting and representing prototypic interactions in that interpersonal world. There is little room for fantasy and there is little evidence of fantasy in these early years, although there is much room for reality-oriented cognition that reflects the infant's and child's level of development and for individual differences in organizing affectively toned experiences.

The capacity for fantasy only appears in the older child. For example, symbolic play only begins to appear at 2 years of age and flourishes at age 3, 4, and 5. I had occasion recently to spend the day with a very bright and imaginative 4-year-old who spent the entire day in play. What struck me about his play was the degree to which every object in reality stood for something else. An ordinary stick became a prince's sword, a towel became a cape, a tarp became a tent, and so on. This sort of play involving imaginative symbolic equivalences is not possible in younger children.

RESEARCH ON ADULT ATTACHMENT PATTERNS

There is evidence supporting Bowlby's (1979) claim that attachment relationships are important "from the cradle to the grave." There is evidence, too, that the availability of one's attachment figure modulates distress not only in infancy and childhood, but also in adulthood. For example, Coan, Schaefer, and Davidson (2006) reported lower threat-related neural activation when married women held their spouse's hand than when holding the hand of a male experimenter. There is also evidence that marital satisfaction, discord, passion, intimacy, and commitment tend to be strongly correlated with self-report questionnaire measures of attachment pattern (Waters, Mernick, Treboux, Crowell, & Albersheim, 2000).

Just as maternal deprivation dysregulates the infant, so similarly does loss of one's attachment figure (usually, one's spouse) in adulthood have dysregulating consequences, as evidenced by greater susceptibility to illness and a higher mortality rate for a period of time following the loss. There is also evidence that, whereas social support is important in other contexts, it does not alleviate the distress of losing one's spouse (Stroebe, Stroebe, Abakoumkin, & Schut, 1996)—a finding that supports Weiss's (1973) distinction between "emotional loneliness" and "social loneliness."

Individual differences in adult attachment patterns are lawfully related to a wide range of areas of functioning. For example, insecure attachment in adolescence, as measured by the AAI, appears to be associated with greater difficulty in successfully negotiating autonomy and separation from parents. Thus, employing the AAI, Bernier, Larose, and Whipple (2005) found that preoccupied adolescents have more difficulty leaving home for college. They show high levels of conflict and need for contact with parents during the transition from home to college. This pattern is not present when the adolescent is not leaving for college, suggesting that separation activates the attachment system and generates the above pattern. Although peer relationships do not usually constitute attachment relationships, there is evidence that attachment security in adolescence and young adulthood is associated with positive friendship qualities, whereas insecure attachment is associated with lack of social skills and interpersonal hostility (e.g., Allen, Porter, McFarland, McElhaney, & Marsh, 2007; Kobak & Sceery, 1988).

The discussion in this chapter has involved a number of issues related to the conceptualization and measurement of individual differences in attachment patterns. The next chapter is devoted to a more direct discussion of how one understands and assesses attachment patterns.

CHAPTER 4

Understanding and Measuring Adult Attachment Patterns

MEASUREMENT ISSUES

As Haydon, Roisman, and Burt (2012) note, "although attachment theory originated as a framework for understanding species-normative developmental adaptation (Bowlby, 1969/1982), the larger focus of relevant empirical research has been on examining the developmental significance of individual differences in attachment-relevant behavior and representations" (p. 591). The attachment research literature has been dominated by studies on individual differences in attachment patterns. Hence, it becomes especially important to understand how attachment patterns are understood and assessed.

The conception and assessment of attachment patterns in infancy, through the Strange Situation, are relatively straightforward and remain relatively close to the fundamentals of attachment theory. That is, the infant's ability to turn to his or her caregiver for comforting when distressed and as a secure base for exploration and play are at the core of attachment classifications in the Strange Situation. Indeed, the availability of the Strange Situation led to an explosion of ecologically valid and productive research on individual differences in infants' attachment patterns. Apparently, there is nothing like the availability of a measurement tool to encourage research in a particular area.

If one wants to investigate individual differences in attachment patterns later in life or if one wants to investigate the hypothesis that attachment patterns established early in life are relatively stable over time, one needs reliable and valid measures of attachment patterns beyond infancy. Thus, if I want to know whether an attachment pattern is stable from time 1 to time 2, I have to be able to employ reliable and ecologically valid measurement tools at both times. However, I can hardly repeat the Strange Situation as an appropriate assessment of attachment pattern in later childhood, adolescence, or adulthood.

The response of the field to the above need has been the development of widely used tools to assess individual differences in adult attachment. (Interestingly, as will be discussed later in the chapter, there are no widely agreed upon tools to measure attachment patterns in middle to late childhood.) As noted in Chapter 2, a major tool, originating in the developmental psychology tradition, is the AAI. The other tool, associated with the social–personality psychology tradition, is the self-report questionnaire, of which the most widely used is the ECR (Brennan, Clark, & Shaver, 1998). The attachment classifications yielded from the AAI and self-report questionnaires show little relationship to each other (Roisman et al., 2007). That is, knowing an individual's classification on the AAI will not help one to predict that individual's classification on the ECR. For someone not very familiar with the attachment literature, this can be very confusing. Which one is *really* measuring attachment pattern, he or she might ask. This chapter addresses the questions of how one understands and measures individual differences in adult attachment patterns. I begin with an examination of the AAI.

WHAT DOES THE AAI MEASURE?

The AAI is a quasi-clinical interview that focuses on the individual's *early experiences with parents*. The attachment classifications yielded by the AAI are based not on the content of the individuals' narrative, but mainly on its *structural properties*. Thus, as noted in Chapter 2, a classification of secure-autonomous will be given to a narrative that is *coherent*—that is, one that is internally consistent with regard to childhood experiences. A narrative that reflects a defensive distancing from early attachment experiences as reflected, for example, in the minimizing of the importance of attachment needs and experiences or that is characterized by inconsistency such as the idealization of parents combined with specific memories that do not support the idealization or even contradict it would be classified as *dismissive*. And finally, a narrative that is marked by vagueness of discourse and evidence of continuing emotional entanglement while reporting early experiences would be classified as *preoccupied*.

The above classifications are based on the assumption that the structural properties of the individual's AAI narratives reflect his or her internal working model of attachment or, as Main, Kaplan, and Cassidy (1985) put it, one's "state of mind" with respect to attachment (p. 68). Thus, a coherent narrative that is characterized by memories of early negative experiences will be as likely to be classified as secure–autonomous (or "earned secure") as a coherent narrative characterized by memories of early positive experiences.

A question that arises here is the relationship between operationally defining security of attachment in terms of such characteristics as narrative coherence and collaborative discourse on the AAI and the conception of security of attachment derived from attachment theory in terms of the individuals' confident expectation of the availability of the attachment figure and his or her ability to use the attachment figure as a safe haven and secure base. Or, to put it another way, in what way does narrative coherence tap into security of attachment as it is defined in attachment theory, namely, use of the attachment figure as a safe haven and secure base and confident expectation in his or her availability? In effect, these questions speak to the validity of the AAI classifications: Do they measure what they are supposed to measure, namely, security of attachment as this concept is defined in attachment theory? As noted, in the Strange Situation, there is a direct, easily discernible relationship between the infants' classification and his or her attachment relevant behavior—turning to mother, being comforted by her, resuming play. This is not the case in the AAI. The relationship between narrative coherence and attachment relevant behavior is not obvious.

What can we say regarding the validity of the AAI? Does it measure what it is supposed to measure? If one focuses on the AAI attachment classifications (i.e., secure–autonomous, dismissive, and preoccupied), it appears that the AAI measures individual differences in security of attachment. And if one interprets these classification labels in terms of attachment theory, one can conclude that, in contrast to secure–autonomous individuals who have a confident expectation in the availability of their attachment figure and are able to use him or her as a secure base (and safe haven), dismissive and preoccupied individuals do not have such an expectation and are deficient in secure base use.

Although that way of understanding the AAI classifications is implied by categories such as secure–autonomous, dismissive, and preoccupied (which parallel the Strange Situation classifications), the fact is that Main et al. (1985) suggest that one can think of AAI narratives in a more nuanced and complex way, as a reflection of the individual's "state of mind with respect to attachment" (p. 68). Thus, a secure–autonomous classification reflects a coherent state of mind, whereas dismissive and preoccupied classifications reflect a relatively incoherent, contradictory, and vague state of mind with respect to attachment.

From a strictly operational perspective, the validity of the AAI classifications is defined by what they are correlated with and what they predict. The AAI established its credentials by demonstrating that mother's AAI classification robustly predicted the attachment status of her infant in the Strange Situation (e.g., Fonagy, Steele, & Steele, 1991). More recently, evidence has emerged indicating that classification on the AAI is predictive of secure base behavior (e.g., seeking and providing support) in adult couples' interaction (Crowell et al., 2002; Wampler, Riggs, & Kimball, 2004). These findings are especially important because they link classification on the AAI narrative to actual "real-life" behavior that plays a central role in attachment theory. As another example of consistency between AAI narratives and attachment relevant behavior in current relationships, Crowell et al. found a substantial correlation ($r = .51$) between security scores obtained from the AAI and CRI.

What is it about the AAI classification that is so robustly predictive of infant attachment status as well as attachment-relevant behavior in adulthood? Or to put it more specifically, why should the coherence of the mother's AAI narrative predict her infant's attachment status in the Strange Situation; and why should an individual's AAI classification predict secure base behavior in adulthood? Before addressing these questions, let me turn to other studies having to do with the validity of the AAI classifications.

PHYSIOLOGICAL AND BEHAVIORAL CORRELATES OF AAI CLASSIFICATIONS

The dismissive classification on the AAI is interpreted as reflecting a state of mind characterized by, among other things, the avoidance or suppression of emotions and memories related to early attachment experiences; the preoccupied classification is understood as reflecting a state of mind characterized by emotional entanglement. These two classifications have been described, respectively, in terms of deactivation and hyperactivation of the attachment system. What is the evidence supporting the hypothesis that dismissive individuals suppress emotions and that preoccupied individuals are overwhelmed by emotions, specifically during the AAI and more generally when interacting in the context of an attachment relationship?

In a seminal study, Dozier and Kobak (1992) reported that dismissive individuals showed increases in electrodermal activity during the AAI. This finding is important because in contrast to other physiological indices (e.g., heart rate), electrodermal activity is viewed as a physiological marker of emotional inhibition. Roisman and his colleagues have built on Dozier and Kobak's work and have investigated the relationship between AAI classifications and physiological, facial expressive, and self-reported emotional responses during the AAI (Roisman, Tsai, & Chiang, 2004). Roisman (2007) also studied the relationship between AAI classifications and physiological responses during the AAI as well as during interactions in marital and premarital couples.

In the first study, Roisman et al. (2004) replicated Dozier and Kobak's (1992) finding of increased electrodermal activity during the AAI for dismissive individuals. This was not found for preoccupied individuals. Rather, preoccupied individuals "showed reliable discrepancies between the valence of their inferred childhood experiences and their facial expressive as well as reported emotion during the AAI" (p. 776). In contrast to both insecure classifications, secure individuals did not show increased electrodermal activity and but did show coherence between the emotional valence of the childhood events they reported and both their facial expressive and self-reported emotional responses.

These findings provide support for the assumption that dismissing individuals do, indeed, suppress their emotional responses when they think and talk about early attachment experiences and in that sense, support the validity of interpreting the dismissive classification on the AAI as a defensive strategy. The findings also support the assumption that preoccupied individuals become emotionally dysregulated when thinking and talking about early experiences, thus lending validity to the interpretation of the preoccupied classification on the AAI as a reflection of continued emotional entanglement in early attachment issues.

In another study, Roisman (2007) obtained physiological responses during the AAI as well as during couples' interactions. He replicated the finding of heightened electrodermal activity of dismissive individuals during the AAI, but also found heightened electrodermal activity for dismissive individuals while they were attempting to resolve conflict with their partner. Although preoccupied individuals showed no consistent pattern of physiological responses during the AAI, they showed increases in heart rate—a sign of physiological activation—while attempting to resolve conflict with their partner. Contrastingly, dismissive individuals show relative incoherence not only in their narratives, but in the disjunction between reports of childhood experiences and physiological responses suggesting inhibition of emotions. These findings parallel reports of avoidant infants showing physiological evidence of distress in response to separation despite seeming not to be distressed (Sroufe & Waters, 1977). As for preoccupied individuals, they show "relative elevated physiological activation in interaction with partners as well as discrepancies between the valence of their inferred childhood experiences and their facial expressive as well as reported emotion during the AAI" (Roisman et al., 2004, p. 776).

The above findings help us understand what the AAI measures. They suggest that "how adults talk about their early memories [in AAI narratives] reflect qualitatively distinct ways in which past experiences with caregivers have been organized intrapsychically" (Roisman et al., 2004, p. 777). Secure individuals show coherence not only in their narratives, but also in the consistency between the emotional valence of their recall of childhood experiences and physiological and expressive responses and reports of experienced emotions.

These findings speak to the construct validity of the AAI classifications and the "nomological network" in which they are embedded. AAI classifications predict a variety of behaviors, for example, infant attachment status, behavior during couples' interactions, and physiological and expressive responses. The question I now turn to is how to understand the predictive ability of the AAI classifications. What are the factors and processes involved? How does one understand the impressive array of behaviors with which the AAI is correlated? Why and in what ways should the relative coherence of one's AAI narrative be linked to security of attachment when the latter is understood in terms of the fundamental criteria of the use of the attachment figure as a secure base and confident expectation of his or her availability? This question is equivalent to asking: What is it that the AAI measures that enables it to predict attachment relevant behaviors?

THE AAI, REFLECTIVE FUNCTION, AND SECURE BASE SCRIPT KNOWLEDGE

I propose that the AAI classifications essentially measure two factors: (1) the individuals' reflective capacity with regard to attachment-relevant representations and (2) his or her knowledge of a secure base script.

Fonagy et al. (1995) have shown that a good deal of the variance on the AAI is accounted for by level of reflective functioning. Thus, a narrative high in reflective functioning is likely to be classified as secure–autonomous. Further, high reflective functioning on the AAI is predictive of the infant's attachment status (Fonagy et al.). If one thinks only in terms of AAI attachment classifications, one would simply conclude that securely attached adults have securely attached infants. However, another possibility is that whether securely or insecurely attached (as defined by attachment theory), caregivers who are able to reflect on their own mental states and those of others (including their infants' mental states) are more likely to be aware of and respond sensitively to their infant and are therefore more likely to have securely attached infants. They are also more likely to be aware of and respond to their adult partners' signals and serve as a safe haven and secure base from their partner. And because they are able to be in touch with and reflect on their own mental states, they are also more likely to use their partner as a safe haven and secure base.

I am suggesting the possibility that one can be high in reflective capacity and have a coherent AAI narrative and nevertheless be insecurely attached when security of attachment is defined as confident expectation in the availability of the attachment figure and secure base use. I am aware of the evidence that attachment classification on the AAI is predictive of secure base behavior and secure base use in adult couples. However, the correlation between the two is not perfect, which leaves room for the possibility that at least some individuals with a high level of reflective capacity and coherent AAI narratives—who are therefore classified as secure–autonomous—do not show a confident expectation in the availability of the attachment figure and a high level of secure base use and secure base behavior.

In contrast to those with low reflective capacity, these individuals are more likely to be aware of their attachment insecurity, more able to reflect on their expectations and representation, and therefore more likely to modify their expectations and representations in the direction of secure attachment. Because of their high level of reflective capacity, as caregivers, these individuals are more likely to function as a safe haven and secure base for their infant—even if they are not securely attached themselves.

Understanding the role of AAI coherence and reflective functioning this way helps one make sense of a number of findings. For example, as noted earlier, Fonagy et al. (1995) reported that high-risk mothers with high reflective functioning are far more likely to have securely attached infants than high-risk mothers with low reflective functioning. AAI coherence and high reflective function notwithstanding, it is difficult to believe that low SES young single mothers living in overcrowded conditions and with difficult and deprived backgrounds have a confident expectation in the availability of their attachment figure and a high level of secure base use. How, then, does one understand Fonagy et al.'s finding? I think the most plausible account is that despite being insecurely attached themselves, these mothers' relatively high level of reflective function enables them to be in touch with their own and their infant's mental states and therefore better able to serve as a safe haven and secure base for their infant. They are better able to keep the "ghosts" out of the nursery. Or, to put it another way, they are better able to reflect rather than repeat.

Consider Levy et al.'s (2006) report that after 1 year of treatment, borderline patients became securely attached as measured by their AAI narratives. Given what we know about borderline personality disorder, it defies plausibility to conclude that these patients are now securely attached in the sense of a confident expectation in the availability of their attachment figure and secure base use. How then does one understand these findings? It is likely that after 1 year of treatment these patients have become more aware and reflective of their "state of mind with respect to attachment"—that is, of their attachment-relevant expectations and representations. This is no small achievement and, as in the case of high-risk mothers, discussed earlier, may influence behavior and attitudes in important ways. Indeed, it may facilitate steps in the direction of achieving "earned secure"[1] attachment. However, to view enhanced coherence and reflective capacity on the AAI as direct measures of secure attachment leads to implausible interpretation of some findings and often overlooks how security of attachment is defined in attachment theory.

AAI CLASSIFICATION AND SECURE BASE SCRIPT KNOWLEDGE

Waters and Waters (2006) and their colleagues have carried out research on what they refer to as secure base script knowledge. As they note, the work in cognitive psychology on scripts and schemas (e.g., Schank & Abelson, 1982) bears a strong family resemblance to Bowlby's (1973) concept of working models (Bretherton, 1987, 1990). They propose "that an individual's history of secure base support is represented in memory as a secure base script" (e.g., Waters & Rodrigues-Doolabh, 2001, p. 187). Accessibility and knowledge of a secure base script mean having it represented as a structure in one's mind. More specifically, it means that based on the history of one's

---

[1] The category "earned secure" is assigned to those individuals who, despite reporting early negative relationship experiences with their caregiver nevertheless present a coherent narrative on the AAI (Main & Goldwyn, 1998; Pearson, Cohn, Cowan, & Cowan, 1994). The assumption is made that these individuals have overcome negative childhood experiences and have been able to achieve a secure state of mind with respect to attachment—hence, the term "earned secure." However, Roisman, Fortuna, and Holland (2006) have presented evidence suggesting that what is referred to as "earned secure" may be due to "mood-related biases in the recall of early experiences" (p. 68). Furthermore, in a prospective study, Roisman, Padrón, Sroufe, and Egeland (2002) found that individuals who report negative early childhood experiences in a coherent manner on the AAI (thus earning a secure attachment categorization) are no more likely to, in fact, have had negative experiences than those who do not report negative early childhood experiences.

experiences, one has internalized the "rule" that one's attachment figure should be available should the need arise. Waters and Waters reason that if secure base support has been consistent in the individual's life history, his or her secure base script should be fully formed and readily accessible in relevant situations. If secure base support has not been consistently available, the individual's secure base script should be more poorly delineated and less accessible. In effect, Waters and Waters equate secure base knowledge and accessibility with secure attachment in the sense of confident expectation in the availability of one's attachment figure. However, it is possible that one may have secure base script knowledge and even have access to this script as an organizing structure without being securely attached, that is, without being confident about the availability of one's attachment figure. It is also possible that secure base script knowledge and accessibility are more important in successfully serving as an attachment figure for another (i.e., one's infant and/or one's partner) than in being able to turn to one's attachment figure as a safe haven and as a secure base. This can be investigated empirically.

Waters and Waters (2006) have developed a means of assessing implicit secure base script knowledge through a prompt-word outline method which consists of the following elements:

1. A story title, for example, "Baby's Morning" or "Doctor's Office."
2. Word sets that pull for and lend themselves to a secure base narrative. For example:

mother	hug	teddy bear
baby	smile	lost
play	stay	found
blanket	pretend	nap

3. A narrative produced by participants that employs the prompt words.

The narratives are then scored on a 7-point scale "indicating the extent to which the passage is organized around the secure base script" (p. 189). Employing this method, Waters and Rodrigues-Doolabh (2001) found that secure base script knowledge as assessed from AAI narratives is highly correlated with AAI narrative coherence ($r = .50$ to $.60$). Furthermore, like the AAI classifications, mother's secure base script knowledge is predictive of her infant's classification in the Strange Situation (Tini, Corcoran, Rodrigues-Doolabh, & Waters, 2003). Most impressive, scores on a secure base knowledge scale taken from the AAI transcripts predicted secure base support and secure base use behavior in a 15-minute couple problem-solving interaction more robustly than AAI coherence (Waters & Brockmeyer, in press).

These findings help explain the AAI's ability to predict a variety of behaviors, including infant attachment status and secure base behavior in infant–mother and adult couples' interactions. A plausible hypothesis is that classification of secure–autonomous on the AAI implicates (1) a high level of reflective functioning with respect to attachment, and (2) a high level of secure base script knowledge and access. Correspondingly, classifications of insecure attachment indicate low levels of reflective functioning and of secure base script knowledge.[2]

These findings on reflective function and secure base script knowledge suggest that at least one main reason mother's AAI classification can predict her infant's attachment status is that a mother high in reflective functioning and in secure base script knowledge is (1) better able to reflect on the mental states of both herself and her infant, and (2) has a more delineated and accessible representation of what it means to function as a secure base.

The question I have posed is whether a high level of reflective function and secure base script knowledge are equivalent to secure attachment in the sense of a confident expectation in the availability of one's attachment figure and one's ability to use the attachment figure as a safe haven and secure base. Is it possible for someone who is insecurely attached herself able to serve as a safe haven and a secure base for her infant (or partner) by virtue of a high level of reflective function and secure base script knowledge? That this might be so is suggested by Fonagy et al.'s (1995) earlier noted finding that a high level of reflective function is especially predictive of her infant's secure attachment status in a high-risk sample of mothers. One can speculate that despite being insecurely attached themselves, a high level of reflective function enables these mothers to better serve as a safe haven and secure base for their infants. To refer to these mothers as "earned secure" seems to me to beg the question insofar as it equates AAI narrative coherence with secure attachment—the very issue that is open to question (see Roisman et al., 2006, on the classification of "earned secure").

In short, it may be the caregiver's reflective capacity and her knowledge of a secure base script rather than her secure attachment status that are instrumental in her infant's attachment status. For those who have had difficult early attachment experiences and may even remain insecurely attached, these capacities and knowledge structures can serve well in not perpetuating the intergenerational transmission of insecure attachment.

---

[2]One limitation of the secure base script method thus far is that it does not distinguish among different insecure classifications.

Perhaps one does not necessarily need to become securely attached oneself in order for one's reflective functioning capacity and secure base script knowledge to have benevolent effects on both one's own life and the lives of one's infant and partner.

In this regard, many attachment-based intervention programs attempt to influence the infant's attachment status not through modifying the caregiver's attachment status, but through enhancing her reflective capacity as well as her knowledge of safe haven and secure base functioning (e.g., Marvin, Cooper, Hoffman, & Powell, 2002). The assumption implicit in these programs is that regardless of the caregiver's attachment status, the infant can benefit from the enhancement of the caregiver's reflective function and secure base script knowledge.

Just as one need not change mother's attachment status in order for an intervention to be effective, Toth, Rogosch, Manly, and Cicchetti (2006) have shown in a study with depressed mothers that effectiveness of the intervention in altering the infant's attachment status was unrelated to the number of mother's depressive episodes. Rather, it was related to enhancing her reflective awareness and, presumably, her behavior.

As noted earlier, equating AAI coherence with secure attachment has led to some difficulty in interpreting findings—for example, the report that borderline patients are scored as securely attached on the AAI after 1 year of treatment (Levy et al., 2006). Given what we know about the difficulty in treating borderline conditions, it is simply not clinically plausible to expect the achievement of secure attachment after 1 year of treatment—when secure attachment is understood in the context of attachment theory.

Operationally, what Levy et al.'s (2006) findings essentially mean is that the borderline patients' AAI narratives have become more coherent. It seems to me that the most plausible interpretation of these data is that, based on their therapeutic experiences, these patients have developed an increased knowledge of a secure base script and an enhancement of reflective function in regard to attachment. These hypotheses can be directly tested.

THE AAI "VERSUS" SELF-REPORT

A good deal of debate has arisen, regarding the validity of self-report versus interview methods of assessing attachment. Although not stated explicitly, the debate often seems to consist of competing claims regarding which instrument "really" measures adult attachment patterns. It makes little sense, however, to ask which measure is really measuring attachment pattern because they are measuring different aspects of attachment. As noted earlier, self-report questionnaires such as the ECR address the individual's conscious attitudes and feelings regarding closeness in *current intimate relationships*; and attachment classifications are arrived at through the *content* of the items endorsed by the individual. Contrastingly, the AAI addresses the individual's reports and memories regarding *early attachment experiences with parents*; and attachment classifications are arrived at not through content, but through structural properties of the individual's narrative.[3]

Perhaps the most productive way to deal with the debate between self report and interview (as well as other non–self-report measures) is to investigate empirically the correlates of each measure. In an important sense, the "meaning" and validity of a measure is determined by its correlates and what it is able to predict. There is evidence, not surprisingly, that AAI and self-report questionnaires are correlated with different variables and different aspects of behavior. As Waters et al. (2002) have shown, AAI classifications are correlated with such variables as infant attachment status, caregiver's provision of secure base support, and caregiver's knowledge of a secure base script, whereas self-report classifications are correlated with such variables as marital satisfaction, marital discord, couples' passion, intimacy, and commitment. As Waters et al. also note, the AAI is generally correlated with narratives and observed behavior, whereas self-report measures are generally correlated with other self-report measures. However, that this is not always the case is shown by Berant, Mikulincer, Shaver, and Segal (2005) finding that self-report measures of attachment are predictive of responses on the projective tests of the Rorschach and Thematic Apperception Test (TAT).

In a recent paper, Haydon, Roisman, Marks, and Fraley (2011) investigated under-researched aspects of the relationship between the AAI and self-report measures of attachment patterns. As noted, there are minimal correlations between AAI and self-report attachment classifications. However, Haydon et al. found significant moderate correlations between negative *inferred experience on the AAI* and self-reported anxiety and avoidant in regard to mother and father. A weaker correlation was found between self-reported anxiety and avoidance in relation to romantic partner on the

---

[3]One of the criticisms that has been directed, particularly by psychodynamically oriented critics, at self-report measures, which would include self-report measures of attachment, is that they do not take into account such factors as self-deception, social desirability, and mainly, defense (e.g., Shedler, Mayman, & Manis, 1993). This failure, the critics claim, results in a misleading picture of the individual's actual functioning.

ECR and negative inferred experience on the AAI in relation to mother, but not in relation to father. It is important to note that (1) when the AAI scale of inferred experiences and the self-report questionnaire focus on the same specific figure (i.e., mother, father), there is greater convergence between the two methods; and (2) when the AAI and self-report tap the same level of response (i.e., content reports of experience), there is greater convergence between the two methods.

Although this chapter is concerned with measurement of adult attachment patterns, I want to comment briefly on measurement in the Strange Situation employing a Principal Components Analysis (PCA). Fraley and Speiker (2003) reported that the behavioral indicators that identify infant's attachment classifications loaded on the two dimensions of attachment avoidance and attachment anxiety. The latent structure found maps quite well onto the avoidance and anxiety dimensions emphasized by self-report methods (Haydon et al., 2011).

Given the above findings, it is now possible to summarize and account for in a coherent way the nature of the differences among the AAI and self-report measures (I will take the ECR as representative of such measures) of attachment patterns:

1. The AAI classifications measure the individuals' implicit and not necessarily consciously available state of mind with respect to early attachment experiences. The ECR measures the individual's consciously available attitudes and feelings toward his or her current romantic partner. There is little agreement between these two measures. Apparently, an individual's conscious reports of attitudes and feelings toward his or her romantic partner tells us little about his or her implicit state of mind with respect to early attachment experiences. It should be no surprise to learn that individuals often do not have access to their implicit representations that are inferred from the structure of their responses.

    If, as argued earlier, level of reflective function and secure base script knowledge account for a good deal of the variance of AAI attachment classifications, it would follow that direct measures of reflective function and secure base script knowledge would be only weakly related to ECR attachment classifications. This can be empirically tested.

2. When the AAI (inferred experiences) and the self-report questionnaires share a common focus on mother and father, as well as a common focus on context of experiences rather than on structure of responses, there is greater convergence between them.

3. It appears that the latent structure of the Strange Situation, the AAI, and the ECR yields two fundamental dimensions of attachment patterns: anxiety and avoidance.

ATTACHMENT PATTERNS AS TRAIT-LIKE OR INTERACTIONAL PHENOMENA

Are attachment patterns best understood as trait-like internal structures or as interpersonal situational phenomena? Some research attention was given to the issue in the context of arguing against the claim that infant attachment patterns largely reflect inborn temperamental differences (e.g., Kagan, 1982, 1995). In an attempt to refute that claim, Sroufe (1985) pointed to evidence that infants can show two different patterns of attachment with two different caregivers (see also Main & Weston, 1981).

On the basis of this and other evidence, Sroufe (1985) and Sroufe and Fleeson (1986) argued that attachment is a "relational construct" and that attachment classifications reflect the history of a particular infant–caregiver dyad. But, as Sroufe observes, Strange Situation classifications, which almost exclusively involve the infant–mother dyad, have been shown to correlate with a wide range of behaviors, including social and cognitive functioning. If, as Sroufe argues, attachment classification can be different for mother and father, the obvious questions are why the particular attachment pattern with the mother is so predictive of these different areas of functioning and which areas of functioning, if any, are predicted by attachment pattern with father.

To complicate matters further, Brussoni, Jeng, Livesley, and MacBeth (2000) have reported a significant genetic contribution to secure and anxious adult attachment, but not to avoidant attachment, suggesting that a response to adverse experiences is more of a factor in avoidant than in anxious attachment. In other words, compared to avoidant attachment, anxious attachment may reflect not only the history of interactions with a particular attachment figure, but also genetic contributions—or, more likely, an interaction between the two, given what we now know about gene activation by experience.

Despite the claim that a given attachment pattern is a relational construct and reflects only the history of a particular relationship or a set of interactions with a particular person, the fact is that much attachment research on individual differences, as well as their measurement, attachment patterns are treated as stable trait-like structures.

Thus, according to Main, Kaplan, and Cassidy (1985), the AAI is designed to measure "the security of attachment in its generality rather than in relation to any particular person or past relationship" (p. 78). Creasey and Ladd (2005) refer to this conception of attachment patterns as "generalized attachment representations" (GARs) (p. 1026). That is, they are viewed as trait-like cross-situational structures. Thus, although the AAI is directed to the individual's early experiences with mother and father, the assumption is that these early experiences become internalized as stable cognitive-affective structures (i.e., working models of attachment) that constitute GARs able to predict concurrent and later attachment-relevant behaviors. Putting it another way, one can say that based on early experiences, the individual develops *generalized* expectations regarding what an attachment figure will and will not do. For example, if an individual's early history is characterized by repeated rejection and neglect, he or she will develop a *generalized* representation and set of expectations regarding attachment figures later in life. As Creasey and Ladd put it, "this person is at risk for the development of an insecure GAR and develops expectancies that they will not receive support when in most need ... they will have developed the expectancy that bad things happen when they experience relationship distress" (p. 1027).

Creasey and Ladd suggest that, in addition to GARs, individuals also develop attachment representations regarding current specific romantic relationships that are tapped by such self-report measures as the ECR. As we have seen, there is little consistency between the individual's GAR (as measured by the AAI) and his or her attachment pattern as measured by self-report. Thus, an individual with a secure GAR may be classified as insecure in a self-report measure and vice versa. In effect, Creasey and Ladd suggest that an individual may show, say, generalized secure attachment and yet be insecurely attached with regard to his or her current romantic partner. Thus, the former is trait-like and the latter is situationally determined. Furthermore, as is generally the case in the relationship between traits "versus" situations, it is the interaction between the two that is most predictive of behavior (Endler & Magnusson, 1976). Similarly, Creasey and Ladd found that although both the AAI and the Relationship Scales Questionnaire (RSQ) yielded main effects in relation to conflict behavior in couples, the most robust results were interaction effects.

With regard to the RSQ, individuals classified as secure on the AAI showed significantly fewer negative tactics, less defensiveness, and less domineering behavior in a couples conflict situation than those classified as insecure. And dismissive and unresolved/insecure individuals showed significantly more negative and domineering behavior than those classified as preoccupied. Most interesting were the findings regarding conflict behavior and the associations between the participants' attachment representations in relation to current partner (on the RSQ) and their GAR (on the AAI). The results indicated that the relationship between avoidant or anxious attachment in regard to current partner and defensive behavior varied with "whether the participant possessed secure or unresolved/insecure generalized attachment representations" (p. 1033). Specifically, individuals who were classified as more secure on the RSQ (or less anxious) and who were also classified as unresolved/insecure on the AAI were more likely to show defensive behavior in couples' conflict situations.

Individuals who had high levels of anxiety on the RSQ were more likely to exhibit contemptuous behavior; however, this was largely attributable to people who were also unresolved/insecure on the AAI. This pattern was especially evident when the participant's partner exhibited negative behavior. Finally, those classified as avoidant on the RSQ were more likely to show domineering behavior when they were also classified as unresolved/insecure on the AAI.

Based on the above and other findings, Creasey and Ladd (2005) concluded that "individuals who are anxious or avoidant about romantic relationships do not necessarily exhibit difficulties if they possess a secure generalized attachment representation" (p. 1035). Even in the face of negative partner behavior, these individuals are less likely to exacerbate the situation by engaging in negative, contemptuous, and domineering behavior themselves. It also works the other way around. That is, individuals with unresolved/insecure GAR showed less negative behavior if they were classified as securely attached in relation to current partner. An interesting question that Creasey and Ladd raise is whether and to what degree the GAR of this latter group could change over time.

The Creasey and Ladd (2005) study sheds much light on the question of whether attachment patterns are best thought of as a situational or a trait construct, as a "relational construct" or an internalized stable structure. One answer to that question that emerged is that it depends on which aspect of attachment behavior one is investigating and measuring. If one is measuring the individual's current relationship with a particular partner, then the attachment classification is obviously a "relational construct," particularly if one assumes that the individual's attachment classification could change were he or she in a different relationship and responding to questionnaire items in regard to the new partner.

What about the view of attachment pattern as a trait-like stable structure? As we have seen, "security of attachment in its generality rather than in relation to any particular person or past relationship" is how Main, Kaplan, and Cassidy (1985) think of AAI attachment classifications. The assumption being made here is that, although like the ECR or other self-report

measures, the AAI also focuses on specific "past relationships" (early experiences with one's mother and father), it nevertheless yields a *generalized*
structure. Embedded in this assumption is the additional assumption that
representations of one's early attachment interactions with one's caregivers
have become internalized as a general stable structure that comes to influence all subsequent attachment relationships. That is, although originating
in specific relationships with mother and father, they now reflect one's general state of mind with respect to all attachment experiences.

The above formulation essentially reflects the fundamental assumption that one's early experiences with caregivers play a special role in shaping one's general state of mind with respect to attachment and influence all
future attachment relationships and representations. One can understand
this quasi-critical period hypothesis as the attachment theory version of the
general psychodynamic assumption that early experiences have a determinative role in shaping personality development.

Although as noted above, it makes a good deal of sense to think of
the ECR as largely situationally determined and the AAI as trait-like, as
Creasey and Ladd (2005) have shown, the two sets of attachment representations interact in influencing behavior. Thus, individuals with generalized
secure attachment are less likely to engage in negative couples behavior
even when they are classified as insecure with regard to their current partner. And individuals with unresolved/insecure generalized attachment, but
who reported more secure representations with current partners, were also
less likely to engage in negative couples behavior. In general then, complex behavior seems to be a product of the interaction between generalized
attachment representations or working models and specific attachment representations or working models in relation to current partner.

It is likely that the two sets of representations or working models can
influence each other. For example, prolonged experience with a rejecting
partner (and a corresponding insecure "situational" representation) may
modify generalized secure attachment in the direction of generalized insecure attachment. Conversely, prolonged experience with an available and
supportive partner may modify generalized insecure attachment representation in the direction of secure attachment. As Creasey and Ladd (2005)
put it, "unresolved/insecure people who begin to trust or feel close to their
partner could be 'works in progress'; the positive perceptions of romantic
relationships and encouraging interactive behavior could possibly help alter
these GAR overtime" (p. 1036).

A belief in the possibility of altering the individual's GAR—at least
partly through interactions with the therapist (i.e., corrective emotional
experiences)—is a linchpin for the practice of psychotherapy (see Chapter
11). In addition, from the perspective of attachment theory, the rigidity

versus susceptibility to change by new experiences can be viewed as an important indicator of degree of psychopathology (see Chapter 10).

The conception of the coexistence of relationship-specific attachment representations and generalized attachment representations (as well as their interaction and mutual influences) raises questions regarding certain formulations of attachment theory, in particular, the assumption that one's attachment pattern (and underlying working model) established early in life (1) remain relatively stable and (2) are likely to characterize later adult attachment relationships. Although these two assumptions tend to be conflated, they are separable ones. Thus, with regard to the first assumption, if one was, say, securely attached as an infant, barring significant environmental changes, one would be likely to be securely attached as an adult. Operationally, this would be seen as stability between attachment classification in the Strange Situation and the AAI.

As for the second assumption, it is possible for one's working model of attachment or GAR to remain stable over time and nevertheless show a relationship-specific attachment pattern that is quite different from one's general state of mind with respect to attachment. For example, one can show stable generalized secure attachment from infancy to adulthood and nevertheless have an insecure representation in regard to one's current attachment relationship. The latter reflects the attachment history of one's current relationship(s)—in particular, the degree to which one's current attachment figure has been available as a safe haven and secure base—which can be different from the history of one's early relationship with caregivers and one's resulting general state of mind with respect to attachment. The very low correlations between the AAI and self-report classifications of attachment, combined with the more robust correlations between the Strange Situation and the AAI attachment classifications (at least in stable environments), suggest that despite the relative stability over time of generalized attachment representations, there is little consistency between these generalized attachment representations and relationship-specific attachment representations.

One can speculate that psychopathology is characterized by a greater degree of consistency between insecure/unresolved generalized attachment representations and relationship specific insecure representations. Contrastingly, one would expect that psychological health is more likely to be characterized by a greater degree of consistency between generalized and relationship-specific secure attachment; or perhaps show a pattern in which at least one attachment representation is secure. The latter suggests that, at least to some degree, attachment representations are open to ongoing experiences. There are various ways of accounting for consistency between generalized and relationship-specific insecure representations. Generalized insecure representations may color or distort current experiences so that even a realistically available attachment may be experienced as unavailable. The individual may select a partner who is likely to be unavailable and thereby confirm his or her GAR. And finally, the individual may pull for responses in his or her partner that will tend to confirm his or her GAR. Of course, all three factors may be at work. These are important areas for future research.

Before leaving the topic of how one conceptualizes attachment patterns, I want to address the distinction between secure base use and secure base behavior and between being able to turn to and use one's attachment figure as a secure base and serving as a secure base oneself. Raising this issue, in effect, constitutes a continuation of the earlier discussion regarding whether one can serve as a secure base (and safe haven) for another, thereby enhancing the other's security of attachment without being securely attached oneself. The robust finding that mother's secure–autonomous classification on the AAI is a potent predictor of her infant's attachment classification in the Strange Situation has generally been interpreted to mean that secure attachment in mother begets secure attachment in infant. One way of interpreting this relationship is that mothers' confident expectation in the availability of her attachment figure, as reflected in her GAR, enables her to better serve as a secure base (and safe haven) for her infant. On this construal, secure base use and serving as a secure base are closely linked. However, there are people who seem able to serve as a secure base (and safe haven) for others, but who are not comfortable with secure base use; that is, there are those who do seem able themselves to turn to others as a secure base (and safe haven). One sees this pattern in adults who were parentified children, in people who repeatedly enact rescue fantasies, and in compulsive caregivers. One also sees people who are "adept" at secure base use, but who seem relatively unable to serve as a secure base. In any case, it seems to me that one needs to distinguish between secure base use and secure base behavior and to differentiate people who are comfortable with both attachment functions from those whose primary emphasis is on only one of these two attachment functions. It would be interesting to determine whether systematic empirical research would support this distinction.

ASSESSMENT OF ATTACHMENT PATTERNS
IN MIDDLE AND LATE CHILDHOOD

As noted earlier, there are no widely agreed upon tools to measure attachment patterns in middle and late childhood. There is no "gold standard" method equivalent to the Strange Situation or the AAI. Rather, there are a multitude of different approaches (partly depending on the age of the child) that include questionnaires (e.g., Kerns, Aspelmeier, Gentzler, & Grabill, 2001); storytelling (e.g., Granot & Mayseless, 2001); narration of autobiographical events (e.g., Ammaniti, Speranza, & Fedele, 2000); family drawings (e.g., Madigan, Goldberg, Moran, & Pederson, 2004); observation of secure base behavior in a separation–reunion paradigm (e.g., Easterbrooks et al., 1993); interview (e.g., Ammaniti et al., 2005); adaptations of the Strange Situation (e.g., Cassidy & Marvin, 1992; Crittenden, 1994; Main & Cassidy, 1988; Marvin, 1977; Schneider-Rosen, 1990); doll play (e.g., Bretherton, Prentiss, & Ridgeway, 1990); and observation of the child's secure base behavior in the home (e.g., Posada et al., 1995; Waters, 1995).

Apart from issues of reliability and validity, an obvious question that arises with regard to the employment of so many different measures is the comparability and degree of agreement among them. As far as I know, no study addresses this question. Without such information it is difficult to evaluate findings of studies that employ different measures of attachment patterns.

One of the conceptual problems in this area is that in contrast to the age periods of infancy and adulthood, attachment theory does not really provide a very clear or widely agreed-upon set of ideas as to what form attachment behaviors and representations should take in middle and late childhood. Simply turning to the core tenets of attachment theory is not very helpful insofar as they have little to say about the developmental aspects of attachment. In this regard, it is interesting to observe, as Kerns (2008) notes, that the first edition of Cassidy and Shaver's *Handbook of Attachment* did not have a chapter on middle and late childhood.

It is as if the implicit assumption were made that insofar as, barring extreme environmental disruptions, attachment patterns established in infancy are especially determinative and will remain stable into adulthood, one need not bother investigating attachment in middle and late childhood. One sees a similar pattern in psychoanalytic developmental theories. There is a great deal of emphasis on Oedipal and pre-Oedipal stages of development, with relatively little attention given to the so-called latency period— as if development were suspended during these years of middle and late childhood.

My impression from the research literature is that attachment status in infancy is perhaps a better predictor of adult attachment pattern than attachment patterns in middle and late childhood. More specifically, although there is some evidence of stability *within* middle and late childhood, there are mixed findings with regard to predicting attachment status in middle and late childhood from attachment status in infancy. For example, Aviezer et al. (2002) reported that infants' attachment status (re: mother) at 1 year of age predicted attachment status (measured by interview) at 11 years of age. However, secure attachment in infancy predicted later *insecure* attachment.

As another example, in a study with a small sample by Ammaniti et al. (2005), there was no significant stability of attachment from ages 1 to 5 to 11. In general, as Solomon and George (1999) note, some studies report high stability from infancy to middle and late childhood, whereas other studies find nonsignificant levels of stability. One of the problems in interpreting these findings is the absence of agreed upon measures of attachment status in middle and late childhood. Without such measures, we do not know whether lack of stability indicates a true shift in attachment or is rather attributable to the nature of the measures employed.

In coming to the end of this chapter, I want to reiterate my impression that the unavailability of "gold standard" measures of attachment statue in middle and late childhood is at least partly attributable to lacunae in attachment theory. As stated earlier, I think that attachment theory provides a clearer conceptual understanding of what secure and insecure attachment look like in infancy and adulthood than what they look like in middle and late childhood. A clearer and more delineated understanding of the developmental trajectory will likely be followed by more adequate measures.

CHAPTER 5

Divergences between Attachment Theory and Early Psychoanalytic Theories

Before discussing specific divergences between attachment and early psychoanalytic theories, I want to take note of overriding and general divergences between the two theoretical perspectives that provide a context for the specific differences. A fundamental assumption of attachment theory is that the main factors that shape the individual's psychological life and that powerfully influence the adequacy of his or her functioning have to do with (1) the degree to which early experiences with one's caregiver(s) have enabled one to develop a sense of security and safety in one's intimate relationships and (2) using that sense of security and safety as a base for comfortably exploring the world and oneself and for developing competencies and skills necessary for optimal functioning. As Bowlby (1980) puts it:

> Intimate attachments to other human beings are the hub around which a person's life revolves, not only when he is an infant or a toddler or a schoolchild but throughout his adolescence and his years of maturity as well, and on into old age. From these intimate attachments a person draws his strength and enjoyment of life and through what he contributes, he gives strength and enjoyment to others. These are matters about which current science and traditional wisdom are at one. (p. 442)

Although Freud would likely have agreed with Bowlby's statement at the level of practical wisdom, the perspective expressed in that statement and reflected in attachment theory is at marked variance with the Freudian emphasis on the gratification and discharge of sexual instinctual drives as central aspects of adequate functioning.

ACTUAL EVENTS VERSUS FANTASY

As noted, a core assumption of attachment theory is that actual events rather than fantasy have a major influence on the development of the infant and child, including their representations. Bowlby's experiences with James Robertson, his work at the London Child Guidance Clinic and residential institutions, his interest in maternal separation and deprivation, and his research for the World Health Organization all sensitized him to the dire effects of negative actual events on the development of the child. These experiences ran quite counter to what he was taught and exposed to in his psychoanalytic training. His own Kleinian analyst, Joan Rivière, wrote in a 1927 paper: "Psychoanalysis is ... not concerned with the real world, nor with the child's or adult's adaptation to the real world, nor with sickness or health, nor virtue or vice. It is concerned simply and solely with the imaginings of the childish mind, the fantasied pleasures and the dreaded retributions" (pp. 376–377). Karen (1994) notes that Bowlby wrote in the margin of his copy of the journal in which Rivière's remarks appeared "Role of environment = zero."

Many years later, Bowlby (1988) recalled: "it was regarded as almost outside the proper interest of an analyst to give systematic attention to a person's real experience" (p. 43). He characterized the standard psychoanalytic view in the following way: "Anyone who places emphasis on what a child's real experiences may have been ... was regarded as pitifully naïve. Almost by definition it was assumed that anyone interested in the external world could not be interested in the internal world, indeed was almost certainly running away from it" (pp. 43–44).

A good example of the tendency to emphasize fantasy over actual events is seen in Bion's reaction to Robertson's film *A Two-Year-Old Goes to Hospital* when it was shown to the British Psychoanalytic Society. In his view the little girl's distress was due to her envy of her mother's pregnancy rather than a reaction to separation (as cited in Holmes, 1995).

Although, as the above quoted passage from Rivière (1927) indicates, there is much justification for the criticism that Klein and Kleinians placed excessive emphasis on fantasy at the expense of attending to actual events in the life of the child, the claim that they totally ignored actual events, at least in their theoretical formulations is not fully justified. Contained in the complex structure of Kleinian theory is the recognition that one needs good objects (i.e., actual good experiences) in order to counteract one's destructive impulses. That is, good object experiences temper and modulate hate, destructiveness, and the death instinct and strengthen love and the life instinct. Tipping the balance in the direction of the latter is necessary if the ego is to survive. As Klein (1975) writes, "preservation of the good object is regarded as synonymous with the survival of the ego" (p. 264). Similarly, Segal (1964) writes that "when there is a predominance of good experience over bad experience, the ego acquires a belief in the prevalence of the ideal object over the persecutory objects, and also the predominance of its own life instinct over its own death instinct" (p. 24). Klein also writes about the importance of reparation to the object because, to quote Klein, it is "such an essential part of the ability to love" (p. 342). In short, although Kleinians do assume that inborn destructive impulses and fantasies play a powerful role in psychological life, at least in their theoretical writings, they do not entirely ignore the influence of actual events.

Despite providing some room for the influence of actual events in the life of the child, Klein and Kleinians not only place great emphasis on fantasy, but also attribute elaborate and complex fantasies to the young infant that seem much beyond his or her capability. Consider two examples taken from Klein's (1975) writings: "It is my experience that in the phantasied attacks on the mother's body a considerable part is played by the urethral and anal sadism which is very soon added to the oral and muscular sadism. In phantasy, the excreta are transformed into dangerous weapons: wetting is regarded as cutting, stabbing, burning, drowning, while the faecal mass is equated with weapons and missiles" (pp. 219–220). As another example, Klein confidently states, "We know that the ejection of the faeces symbolizes a forcible ejection of the incorporated object and is accompanied by feelings of hostility and cruelty and by destructive desires of various kinds, the buttocks receiving importance as an object of these activities" (p. 253). What is one to make of such passages! There is certainly no good evidence for such fantasies, and it is difficult to imagine how such evidence could be obtained. Rather, claims regarding the existence of these fantasies are based on mere assertion and speculation and on so-called reconstruction from the productions of adult patients in treatment.

One charitable—perhaps too charitable—interpretation of Rivière's remarks is that she was not denying the impact of actual events on the life of the child, but was stating that the bailiwick of psychoanalysis was not the events themselves, but the meaning given to these events. That is to say, psychoanalysis is concerned with *psychic reality*. When viewed this way, the issue between attachment theory and psychoanalysis is no longer one of actual events versus fantasy, but rather one of the relationship between actual events and psychic reality—or, to put it another way, the relationship between actual events, on the one hand, and how these events are experienced, the meanings given to them, on the other hand. This, I believe, is a legitimate issue that both makes clinical sense and that is, in principle, susceptible to empirical investigation.

As we have seen in Chapter 3, there is a lawful relationship between independent judgments of maternal sensitivity and responsiveness and the infant's attachment pattern, which suggests that the infant's internal working model of the caregiver and interactions with her are reasonably accurate. However, although lawful, as noted, the relationship between infant's attachment pattern (and the internal working model underlying it) and maternal responsiveness and sensitivity is a modest one. To a certain extent, this may be due to "noise" and errors of measurement. However, the modest size of the relationship also suggests that other factors may be at work, among which may be how the child experiences the caregiver's behavior.

Let me take the liberty of quoting a long passage from my paper on attachment and psychoanalysis (Eagle, 1997):

> Although this is ultimately an empirical question, for a number of reasons, it seems unlikely that there would be a direct and simple relationship between attachment style and internal working model, on the one hand, and actual behavior of the caregiver, on the other. For one, the child's immature cognitive capacities, conflicts, wishes, and fantasies could generate distortions in his or her perception and understanding of the caregiver's behavior. But perhaps most important, given individual differences among infants in constitution and temperament, expressed in such specific dimensions as soothability, irritability, and frustration tolerance, it seems inevitable that different infants will experience the caregiver's behavior in idiosyncratic ways. For example, one infant may react to a short delay in being fed with equanimity, whereas another infant may become more frustrated and enraged. Similar or identical caregiving behavior may be experienced differently and therefore represented and encoded differently by different infants. If this is so, it would suggest that internal working models and other representations could not be entirely veridical in the sense of corresponding directly to actual events in any simple way. Rather, they would necessarily bear the mark of the individual's idiosyncratic way of experiencing the world. (p. 218)

Thus, the psychoanalysts' criticism that attachment theory tends to deemphasize psychic reality may be partly justified. One of Bowlby's main goals in his development of attachment theory was to demonstrate that infants are powerfully affected by loss and separation and that early experiences of deprivation and rejection have a lasting influence. In the language of statistics and research design, one can say that Bowlby was interested primarily in demonstrating main effects rather than interaction effects. That is, he wanted to demonstrate that environmental and causal factors A, B, and C (i.e., separation, loss, threats of separation, rejection) are lawfully related to effects D, E, and F (e.g., delinquency, mourning, depression). He was less concerned with qualifying that relationship by the observation that A, B, and C have causal effects D, E, and F only if or mainly if factors G, H, and I (e.g., the meaning given to these events, the presence of other supports) also obtain. Also, perhaps Bowlby was not especially interested in interaction effects because he assumed that loss, separation, and the like have such powerful main effects that they would dwarf or render insignificant any qualifying interaction effects.

One of the problems, particularly for the researcher and theorist, with an emphasis on the idiosyncratic meaning given to events, that is, on psychic reality, is that it immediately raises the question of what determines differences in psychic reality. If the impact of environmental events on development is a function of the meanings given to these events, surely, an adequate and comprehensive theory of personality would include an account of the factors that influence the meanings given, that is, that influence psychic reality. This is not a particularly pressing issue for the clinician who wants to understand and perhaps alter these meanings rather than uncover, in the philosopher Max Black's (1967) words, their "provenance and etiology" (p. 656). However, it is a critical issue for the researcher and theorist whose aim is to develop an adequate theory accounting for the relationship between particular sets of early experiences and particular aspects of later development. Although the individual's psychic reality will constitute a partial explanatory account that may suffice for clinical purposes and at the level of folk psychology (Stich, 1983)—for example, event X has effect Y because it is given meaning Z—in a comprehensive theory, the meanings given to an event constitute phenomena that themselves need to be explained (i.e., which factors determine the meanings given to events).

There is little doubt that actual events such as separation, loss, abuse, and so on may have profound and lasting effects on development. That is hardly a debatable issue. However, there is evidence that the impact of these events and how the child experiences them may interact with other factors such as the presence of a supportive figure and the arrangements made for the child following the traumatic events (e.g., Rutter, 1976). Of course, these other factors are also actual events rather than endogenous fantasies. However, other factors that influence the impact of actual events may include temperamental differences and the child's immature level of cognition. For example, a young child may experience a caregiver's behavior as rejection when, in fact, it may be due to depression or illness or fatigue.

MULTIPLE WORKING MODELS

A sharp dichotomy between actual events and fantasy is not tenable even from the perspective of attachment theory. As noted, Bowlby (1973) writes that "the particular form that a person's working models take are a fair reflection of the types of experience he has had in his relationships with attachment figures" (p. 297). This is a straightforward claim that working model representations constitute a relatively accurate reflection of actual events. However, Bowlby also allows for the possibility of multiple internal working models, one relatively accessible to consciousness and one "relatively or completely unconscious" (p. 239), that may conflict with each other. It is clear that Bowlby views the unconscious working model as an accurate representation of actual events in contrast to the conscious working model which is often the distorted product of defense.

A good example of multiple internal working models is seen in the avoidant attachment pattern. Whereas the infant's overt behavior may suggest that he or she does not need mother as a safe haven for comforting and a secure base for exploration, physiological indices such as cortisol secretion and heart rate acceleration suggest otherwise. The presence of conflicting and contradictory working models in adulthood is seen in the avoidant individual's idealization of parents on the AAI, combined with concrete examples that contradict the idealized representation or the individual's inability to provide any concrete memories that instantiate the idealized pictures. The understanding of this pattern is that the conscious idealized representation is the product of defense and masks an unconscious working model of parental figures as rejecting and of oneself as unworthy of love. In short, even from the perspective of attachment theory, the claim that "working models are a fair reflection ... " is no longer tenable in any simple or straightforward way. Indeed, the idealization characteristic of avoidant attachment can serve as a good example, not only of defense, but of the use of fantasy in the service of defense.

Whereas the hypothesis of multiple working models in conflict with each other seems to be a plausible one with regard to avoidant attachment, it does not appear to work as well in relation to anxious attachment or enmeshed/preoccupied attachment. Thus, in the case of avoidant attachment, conscious idealization of parents is understood as a defense against memories and feelings linked to early experiences of rejection—which, in Bowlby's (1980) words are dealt with through "exclusion of information from further processing" (p. 44). What is the nature of the unconscious working model, the awareness of which is defended against and that is in conflict with the conscious working model in the case of anxious attachment? Does the anxiously attached individual ward off memories and experiences of inconsistent caregiving analogous to the avoidant's "defensive exclusion" of memories and experiences of rejection? The answers to these questions do not seem evident. Whereas avoidant attachment seems clearly to entail defenses and lends itself to a formulation in terms of multiple working models and the attachment theory version of a "dynamic unconscious," this is not apparent in the case of anxious attachment. (Recall the discussion in Chapter 2 of anxious attachment, which is seen as much a failure of defense as a relatively intact operational defense.)

CONCEPTIONS OF UNCONSCIOUS PROCESSES

Bowlby (1973) writes that "the hypothesis of multiple models, one of which is highly influential but relatively or completely unconscious is no more than a version, in different terms, of Freud's hypothesis of a dynamic unconscious" (p. 239). Bowlby's comment notwithstanding, the differences between his and Freud's conception of a dynamic unconscious are not simply a matter of "different terms." Bowlby's dynamic unconscious is one of representations of interactions and experiences, whereas Freud's dynamic unconscious is one of repressed wishes and fantasies linked to sexual and aggressive drives—a "cauldron full of seething excitations" (Freud, 1933/1964, p. 73).

As we will see in Chapter 6, this very divergence between attachment theory and classical psychoanalysis with regard to the nature of the "dynamic unconscious" constitutes points of convergence between attachment theory and contemporary conceptions of mind in terms of "transactional patterns" (Mitchell, 1988, p. 17).

THE BASIS FOR INFANT–CAREGIVER ATTACHMENT

A major theoretical impetus for the development of attachment theory lay in Bowlby's rejection of the Freudian secondary drive theory account of the basis of the infant's attachment to his or her caregiver and his insistence that attachment was based on an autonomous inborn behavioral system.

According to secondary drive theory, the infant develops an attachment to the caregiver because she is associated with reduction of the infant's hunger drive. Thus, the caregiver takes on secondary reinforcing properties. This view was held not only by Sigmund Freud and Anna Freud, but also by the learning theorist Clark Hull (e.g., 1943, 1951) who exerted a great deal of influence on academic psychology in the 1940s and 1950s. In this view, there are a limited number of so-called primary drives, such as hunger and sex, that energize behavior; and it is stimuli associated with the reduction of these drive tensions that take on secondary reinforcing properties. This was the dominant theory held by Freudians and the tension-reduction or drive-reduction learning theorists who flourished in the 1940s and 1950s. Although it may be difficult to imagine today, the tension-reduction behavioral learning theorists viewed aspects of Freudian theory as highly congruent with their own views. Indeed, one of Hull's earliest papers was on Freudian theory. And in a book that was quite influential at the time, Dollard and Miller (1950), two neo-Hullians, presented a systematic translation of Freudian concepts into Hullian learning theory terms.

This was the theoretical orthodoxy that seemed wrong-headed, not only to Bowlby, but also to others, foremost among whom was the prominent researcher, Harry Harlow. In what is perhaps the most well-known experiment in the history of psychology, Harlow (1958) demonstrated that reduction of hunger in infant monkeys did not serve as a primary basis for attachment. Rather than becoming attached to the surrogate wire "mother" who provided milk, monkeys became attached to the surrogate terrycloth "mother" who provided "contact comfort." Harlow's study came pretty close to constituting a crucial experiment that definitively refuted an opposing theoretical account. However, compatible with the views of Lakatos (1978) on theory change, Hullian tension-reduction theory was already tottering due to the sheer weight of evidence against it. (See the work of the early cognitivists, such as Tolman [e.g., 1948].) Harlow's findings dealt the final blow.

Bowlby was aware of and welcomed Harlow's findings, which were in accord with his contention that infant–mother attachment was not based on hunger reduction. However, it should be noted that Harlow's findings are not especially relevant to the idea of an inborn autonomous attachment system. They can be plausibly interpreted as evidence for a new version of a secondary reinforcement model—a non-drive reduction one—of infant–caregiver attachment. That is, if one posits a primary need for "contact comfort," as Harlow does, one can say that the infant monkey becomes attached to its caregiver because of her association with "contact comfort."

This may not be a drive-reduction secondary reinforcement model, but it is a secondary reinforcement model of some kind (see Chapter 7).

It seems to me that one needs to distinguish between two claims that can become conflated. One claim, which in certain respects, is at the heart of attachment theory, is that the attachment system is selected for as a primary and an autonomous system that is not secondarily derived from other presumably more primary systems (e.g., hunger and feeding). In short, there is an inborn tendency to become attached. This claim bears a strong family resemblance, in the psychoanalytic context, to Fairbairn's (1952) insistence that "libido is primarily object-seeking" (p. 82). The second claim has to do with the factors that determine the *specific figure* to whom the infant becomes attached rather than the origins of attachment itself. Harlow's findings have to do with this second claim rather than the first. They appear to demonstrate that tactile stimulation rather than feeding constitutes a stronger basis for determining to whom the infant monkey becomes attached (more on this in Chapter 7).

To sum up, all the evidence taken together appears to strongly support Bowlby's proposals that (1) attachment is an inborn autonomous system, and (2) that the specific figure to whom the infant becomes attached is not primarily determined by reduction of the hunger drive. As we will see in Chapter 7, there is a good deal more to say regarding the factors that determine the specific figure to whom the infant becomes attached.

THE OEDIPAL PERIOD VERSUS EARLIER EXPERIENCES: TRIANGLES VERSUS DYADS

Whereas according to Freudian theory, the vicissitudes of the Oedipal period play a determinative role in personality development, the focus of much attachment research is on the first year or two of life. An overwhelming number of studies on attachment patterns—exploiting the availability of the Strange Situation as a research tool—are concerned with the first year to year and a half of the child's life. This focus is consistent with the hypothesis that internal working models are formed quite early in life and subsequently are relatively resistant to change.

That attachment and Freudian theories are concerned with different developmental periods is not fortuitous, but is inherent in the phenomena in which they are primarily interested. Insofar as attachment theory is especially concerned with the infant–mother attachment, it will, of course, focus on the earliest period of life and on the infant–mother dyad. Similarly, insofar as Freudian theory is concerned primarily with sexuality and aggression, it will focus on the Oedipal period, which presumably marks the culmination of infantile sexuality and the introduction of triangularity into psychic life.

In this regard, it is not surprising to observe that attachment theory has virtually nothing to say about the role of triangular relationships in psychological development. This observation serves as a reminder that attachment theory is not intended to cover and account for all aspects of development and psychic life. However, I believe that Bowlby's apparent lack of attention to triangularity was not only due to his focus on the development of attachment theory, but may also be attributable to his skepticism about the claim that the vicissitudes of Oedipal conflicts play a major role in psychological development.

Contrary to the determinative role that Freud gave to infantile sexuality and Oedipal conflicts, Bowlby believed that it was the impact of early attachment-related experiences of separation, rejection, and so on, that played a major role in the development of personality, including the etiology of psychopathology. This divergence from Freudian theory is not a matter of stressing the so-called pre-Oedipal along with Oedipal factors. It is rather a matter of denying that Oedipal factors have the great influence that is attributed to them in Freudian theory.

METHODOLOGICAL DIVERGENCES

The divergences between attachment theory and psychoanalysis are not limited to the content of the different theories, but extend to methodological and epistemological differences regarding the acquisition of evidence that forms the basis for these theories. Thus, as Fonagy (2001) puts it, Freud's speculations about the infant's earliest period of life were "abstract, fictional, and not based on direct observation" (p. 51). Although many psychoanalytic institutes require a course on infant observation, it is not at all clear that this requirement has had any impact on psychoanalytic theorizing about infancy. Further, many psychoanalytic formulations regarding the influence of early experiences on personality development are not primarily based on data emerging from direct observation, let alone longitudinal studies. Rather, they are frequently based on "reconstructive" inferences from work with adult patients (see Chapter 7). Although "reconstructions" or, as Freud (1937b/1964) proposed, constructions in the analytic situation may be useful clinically, they can hardly serve as reliable data for theoretical formulations regarding the nature of infant and child development.

The psychoanalytic dismissal of extraclinical data has a long and hallowed tradition that goes as far back as Freud's response to Rozenweig (1934) who informed him of some experimental support for a psychoanalytic formulation to the effect that while the results were interesting and could do no harm, they were already known by psychoanalysts (cited in MacKinnon & Dukes, 1964). In short, a methodological and epistemological clash was there from early on and continues to the present day between the empirical research focus of attachment theory as well as its appeal to nonpsychoanalytic evidence (e.g., ethological findings) and the psychoanalytic tradition of basing its theoretical formulations almost exclusively on inferences and speculations from clinical data generated in the psychoanalytic situation.

The clash is an understandable one insofar as attachment theory is strongly associated with a systematic research program largely carried out in university settings, whereas most psychoanalysts are engaged in clinical work (the great majority of them in clinical work with adults). For the latter, the primary focus is on treating people, and the primary means of, so to speak, obtaining data is through the clinical encounter, not through carrying out research. Given the "mandate" to treat people, the clinician is more concerned with whether an inference or so-called reconstruction regarding the influence of early experience is therapeutically helpful rather than veridical. Thus, what is important to at least some clinicians is whether a narrative is persuasive and mutative (which Spence, 1982, unfortunately refers to as "narrative truth") rather than whether it is accurate. The researcher, on the other hand, is devoted to investigating lawful relationships, for example, between early experiences and later development. For the developmental researcher the "gold standard' is longitudinal studies that yield reliable predictions. Contrastingly, as Freud and others have noted, in its clinical guise, psychoanalytic accounts are necessarily retrospective rather than prospective. Their purpose is therapeutic impact rather than etiological prediction.

Many clinicians view the general findings and categories (e.g., different attachment patterns) that emerge from research programs as perhaps interesting, but not very useful in providing richly textured idiosyncratic descriptions required by clinical work with individual patients. Or so the argument goes. This methodological divergence between psychoanalysis and attachment theory is based not only on the content of the different theories, but also on the clash between clinician and researcher (see Eagle & Wolitzky, 2011; Hoffman, 2009).

A final divergence between attachment theory and early psychoanalysis I want to note is one between what one may refer to as the metapsychologies of Freud and attachment theory. Bowlby (1969/1982) makes clear that although he has no difficulty accepting the structural, genetic, and adaptive point of view, he cannot accept either Freud's "psychical energy model" and his central idea that the basic function of mind is to discharge excitation or his view of psychological functioning in terms of buildup and discharge of excitation. Bowlby notes that in adopting a psychical energy model, Freud was borrowing from the reliance on energy concepts of the science of his day. He also notes that, similar to Freudian theory, attachment theory is also borrowing from its contemporary scientific climate. In particular, the model of instinctive behavior proposed by attachment theory borrows from ethology, work in behavioral systems and their control, information theory, and an understanding of homeostatic systems. Finally, Bowlby makes clear that although attachment theory "derives from object-relations theory" (p. 17), what distinguishes it from object relations theory is that, like Freudian theory, it provides a model of instinctive behavior. For Bowlby, embedding a theory of human behavior in biology and evolutionary theory was essential.

CHAPTER 6

Divergences between Attachment Theory and Later Psychoanalytic Theories

The later psychoanalytic theories of object relations theory, self psychology, relational psychoanalysis, and intersubjective theory reject Freudian drive theory, place greater emphasis on actual early events (e.g., love vs. rejection, empathic understanding vs. lack of it), and stress relational and interactional factors. To the extent that they share this perspective with attachment theory, one would expect fewer divergences and greater points of convergence between these theories and attachment theory. Indeed, that is generally the case. However, there remain significant points of divergence between attachment theory and these later psychoanalytic theories.

METHODOLOGICAL DIVERGENCES

The clash of methods and attitudes between attachment theory and psychoanalysis that are linked to the different perspectives of researchers and clinicians discussed in the previous chapter applies equally to contemporary psychoanalytic theories. Object relations, self psychology, relational, and intersubjective psychoanalysts are generally no more likely to refer to empirical studies in their writing and formulations than Freudian or Kleinian analysts. Hoffman's (2009) plenary address at the winter meetings of the American Psychoanalytic Association referred to systematic empirical research as entailing the "dessication of human experience" and constituting "doublethinking our way to scientific legitimacy." He received a standing ovation from analysts of presumably different theoretical orientations.

In a 1998 paper, Mitchell, the leading figure of relational psychoanalysis, satirically refers to a "clinical state that I have to come to think of as the Grunbaum syndrome. ... What follows for an analyst afflicted with the Grunbaum syndrome is several days of guilty anguish for not having involved oneself in analytic research. ... However, it invariably passes in a day or so and the patient is able to return to a fully productive life" (p. 5). So much for grappling with issues of research, methodology, and evidence (see Eagle, Wolitzky, & Wakefield, 2001)!

This general methodological divergence remains and is quite apparent in recent discussions of the role of infant observation in psychoanalysis. "Reconstructive" inferences about infancy are defended by some as generating reliable evidence regarding the nature of infant experience.[1] For example, Green (2000) contrasts the "real" child of direct observation with the "true" child of psychoanalysis, suggesting that both have equal probative value.

In making this distinction, Green's interest is in making inferences regarding the presumed "residues" of childhood experiences and fantasies as they presumably appear in the productions of adult patients in analytic treatment rather than formulating a theory of child development. This intention is obscured, however, by the use of the terms "real" child and "true" child, which gives one the misleading impression that the inferences from the data of direct observation of the child and from the adult patient's productions in analytic treatment have equal standing in formulating a theory of child development.

Green (2000) argues that infant research is not particularly relevant for carrying out psychoanalytic treatment with adults. That may or may not be the case—although I am inclined to agree with Green. However, it is entirely untenable to maintain that inferential reconstructions from adult patients' reports and free associations constitute reliable data regarding childhood experiences or that such inferential reconstructions somehow

---

[1]There are important exceptions to this trend in the work of such individuals as Emde, Fraiberg, Greenspan, Lieberman, Mahler, Pine, and Stern. However, with the exception of Mahler, this work does not appear to have markedly influenced the main psychoanalytic theories of infancy and child development.

represent the "true" child (of psychoanalysis).[2] In fact, although one may focus on different aspects of the child's experiences and take different perspectives on childhood experiences and development, there is only one child; and one learns about that child by interacting with and observing him or her.

The inclusion of infant observation as a required course in some psychoanalytic institutes suggests an increasing awareness of the limitations of inferential reconstructions. It is not clear, however, that this requirement has had much of an impact on psychoanalytic theorizing about infancy. Consider the fact that Kohut's (1984) etiological theorizing on the effects of the lack of early parental mirroring on the development of self-defects and narcissistic personality disorder does not include a single reference to an empirical study investigating this relationship. There may, indeed, be empirical support for this formulation. But the points are (1) that Kohut did not see the necessity of citing such evidence and (2) that institutes that include courses on self psychology present Kohut's hypothesis as canonical and are not likely to refer to this gap in Kohut's theorizing.[3]

I recall giving a paper at a psychoanalytic institute on attachment and sexuality (which will be discussed in Chapter 8). In discussing Oedipal conflicts and in weighing the evidence for the hypothesis of universal incestuous wishes, that paper also included some reference to animal research. During the discussion period, the first comment made from the floor was that my paper did not take a "psychoanalytic perspective." The point here is not whether or the degree to which my paper took a "psychoanalytic perspective," but rather that this should be of primary concern, indeed, of greater concern than weighing the evidence—from whatever source—in evaluating the tenability of a particular theoretical formulation. In short, the "bad blood" between attachment theory and psychoanalysis to which Fonagy (2001) refers has as much to do with a clash in epistemological attitudes and values as with the content of competing theories.

Let me now turn to more specific divergences between attachment theory and later psychoanalytic theories. Fonagy (2001) has already provided an excellent summary account of these divergences. My comments in this

---

[2] Just as one cannot construct an adequate theory of child development based on data from adult patients in treatment, so similarly, one cannot construct an adequate theory of adult treatment based on data from observations of infants or infant–caregiver dyads (a project attempted by Beebe & Lachmann, 2002). At best, one can find evocative analogies.

[3] I refer to self psychology as illustrative. The same points can be made with regard to other "schools" of psychoanalysis.

chapter will be limited to selective issues that, I believe, merit further comment.

ATTACHMENT THEORY AND SELF PSYCHOLOGY

Self psychology views empathic understanding and attunement as essential components of healthy psychological development. This is generally compatible with the emphasis in attachment theory on the importance of maternal sensitivity and responsiveness. However, there are also a number of significant divergences between the two theoretical perspectives.

1. Although central to self-psychology theory, the concept of self-cohesiveness plays little or no role in attachment theory.

2. Whereas from a self-psychology perspective, the primary consequences of traumatic parental failures in providing empathic understanding are self defects and narcissistic personality disorder, the consequences of lack of maternal sensitivity and responsiveness identified in attachment theory and research are insecure patterns of attachment. Furthermore, whereas self-defects and narcissistic personality disorders are forms of pathology, insecure patterns of attachment are not in themselves expressions of pathology, but rather may constitute risk factors for pathology.

3. Self defects are largely "automatic" consequences—in a rather linear cause and effect way—of early environmental failures in empathic mirroring and opportunities for idealization. In contrast, in attachment theory, insecure patterns of attachment are understood as *defensive and coping strategies* for dealing with various forms of parental behavior.[4] Implicit in the latter view is the idea that the risk of pathology will be a function of a number of factors such as rigidity of attachment patterns, dimensional issues such as how avoidant or anxious the individual is, and interaction of attachment pattern with other factors.

4. Self psychology locates therapeutic action in the therapist's empathic understanding and the empathic bond between therapist and patient—a form of corrective emotional experience, as acknowledged by Kohut (1984). According to Bowlby's (1988) conception of the therapeutic situation, the therapist serves as a secure base from which the patient can engage in self-exploration. As Bowlby puts it, one of the main functions of the therapist "is to provide the patient with a secure base from which he can explore the

---

[4]Kohut does refer to compensatory and defensive strategies.

various unhappy and painful aspects of his life, past and present, many of which he finds it difficult or perhaps impossible to think about, reconsider without a trusted companion to provide support, encouragement, sympathy, and, on occasion guidance" (p. 138). Although Bowlby does refer to the positive impact of the therapeutic relationship itself, the above passage suggests that for Bowlby, therapeutic action resides equally in the self-exploration facilitated by the availability of a secure base.

Mace and Margison (1997) write that there has been a tension in the attachment literature between a "cognitive effort towards understanding of the unsatisfactory working model and a fundamental attempt to offer rehabilitation through a positive attachment experience" (p. 213). However, it seems to me that the emphasis in the attachment literature has been on the former. Thus, it is no accident that Fonagy and his colleagues (e.g., Allen, Fonagy, & Bateman, 2008; Fonagy, Bateman, & Luyten, 2012) identify attachment theory as the theoretical context for the overriding importance given to mentalization and reflective function. In this regard, Bowlby's conception of the effective ingredients in treatment is closer to the traditional emphasis on self-awareness and self-reflection than it is to the self-psychology perspective. Indeed, Kohut (1984) makes it clear that expansion of self-awareness is not an essential goal of treatment from a self-psychology perspective, whereas self-exploration and the enhanced awareness it generates is central to the attachment theory conception of treatment goals.

5. Whereas Kohut (1984) places much importance on the necessity of idealization of parental figure and "twinship" experiences in healthy development, these factors play no role in the conception of optimal development in attachment theory. Indeed, at least in adulthood, idealization of parents on the AAI is associated with insecure attachment. However, we do not know whether idealization in childhood—Kohut's focus—is associated with optimal development.

ATTACHMENT THEORY AND OBJECT RELATIONS THEORY

I focus mainly on Fairbairn's formulations insofar as they constitute the most systematic articulation of object relations theory. Although in certain respects, attachment theory can be understood as one variant of a broad object relations theory perspective, there are, nevertheless, significant points of divergence between the two.

1. Bowlby (1969/1982) noted that Fairbairn's formulations do not contain a biological instinct theory. This, for Bowlby is a significant weakness

given his biological evolutionary perspective. To say, as Fairbairn (1952) does, that "libido is primarily object-seeking" (p. 82) does imply an inborn basis for object relations, but does not place that tendency in a broader biopsychological evolutionary context.

2. Both Bowlby and Fairbairn emphasize the role of actual early events of rejection and deprivation in the development of maladaptive representations, including maladaptive self-representations. However, they have very different ways of accounting for the processes through which these representations develop and how they function in the personality. For Fairbairn, the effects of early rejection and deprivation include the internalization of "bad" objects. That is, the rejecting and depriving other—one should say the attitudes and valuations of the other—become internalized as part of one's personality structure.[5] In Fairbairn's (1952) words, an "internal saboteur" is now lodged in the personality.[6] The result is "splits in the ego" or inner conflict in which one's needs and wishes for emotional nurturance and love are met with one's own critical and demeaning attitude.

We know that Bowlby's concept of internal working model can also include representations of oneself as unworthy and undeserving of love and nurturance. However, in attachment theory, such representations are largely the product of relatively straightforward learning, whereas in Fairbairn's object relations theory, they are defensively motivated in at least two ways: (a) internalizing the object sustains the child's fantasy of controlling it and (b) viewing oneself, rather than the object as "bad" and unworthy, keeps alive the hope that if one is "good" love may be forthcoming. In other words, conditional rejection, with the possibility of redemption is far preferable to unconditional rejection. To quote Fairbairn (1952) again, "it is better to live as a sinner in a world ruled by God than to live in a world ruled by the devil" (pp. 66–67). Viewing oneself as "bad," Fairbairn tells us, helps the child keep alive the hope that if one is "good" and worthy, one will earn the object's love. To be rejected and unloved when one is "good" is to experience unconditional rejection.

There is another subtle but important difference between the concepts of internal working model and internalized object-relational representations.

---

[5]This aspect of Fairbairn's theorizing is similar to Sullivan's (1953) idea that the self develops through "reflected appraisals of significant other."

[6]As Fairbairn (1952) notes, the model for his concept of internalized object is Freud's concept of the superego. Both have in common the idea of the internalization of external attitudes that now function as internal critics.

As noted, according to the former perspective, one's representation of one-self as unworthy is a product of learning. According to Fairbairn, one's representation of oneself as unworthy is one aspect of the personality (i.e., antilibidinal ego–rejecting object) that is in dynamic conflict with another aspect of the personality that continues to pursue love and nurturance (i.e., the libidinal ego–accepting object).

One way to articulate these differences is to say that according to attachment theory the main clinical issue is that, based on repeated rejection from the caregiver, one comes to view oneself as unworthy of love from the other. According to Fairbairn's formulations, the main clinical issue is that, also based on repeated rejection, the patient develops active and ongoing contempt for his or her own needs for love and nurturance. It is one thing to view oneself as unworthy of love and nurturance, while continuing to value them as desiderata. It is another thing to experience the need for love and nurturance themselves as contemptible and indications of repulsive weakness. These different views suggest somewhat different therapeutic foci: alteration of internal working models according to an attachment theory perspective versus, in Fairbairn's (1952) phrase, "dissolution of the cathexis of bad objects" (p. 74).

3. Both Fairbairn's object relations theory and attachment theory stress the maintenance and persistence of maladaptive representations and modes of relating. However, Bowlby says little about the maintenance and persistence of these representations (internal working models) beyond the general statement that structures, once formed, are relatively resistant to change (an assumption in accord with Rapaport's [1967, p. 891] conception of structure as being self-sustaining).

Fairbairn has a more dynamic model of the maintenance and persistence, not only of early modes of relating, but also of what may underlie these early modes of relating, namely, the persistence of early object ties. Fairbairn (1952) proposes that patients often show a "devotion" and "obstinate attachment" to early objects such that altering early modes of relating and loosening early object ties are equivalent to abandoning and betraying these early figures. This in turn elicits guilt associated with imagined abandonment and the terror of living in an empty inner world devoid of vital emotional ties to objects.

Some years ago I treated a Canadian Indian man whose pattern of behavior seemed to illustrate the kind of "devotion" to early objects described by Fairbairn. This young man had a history of periods of self-destructive behavior, including drinking sprees accompanied by quasi-suicidal actions such as speeding and, on one occasion, falling into a drunken sleep outdoors throughout a cold, wintry night in Toronto. Quite unusual, given his background, this young man had earned a master's degree in English and was a talented poet, as attested to by a number of published poems that had been quite well received. However, his experience of any success and good fortune (e.g., some sense of relative well-being, a decent job, a poem accepted for publication) was invariably followed by self-destructive behavior and an exacerbation of depression and/or rage.

What was most striking about this patient was the degree to which achievement of success in what he referred to as the white man's world was experienced, in a very profound way, as a betrayal of his own world, his own background, and his own people. The patient's miserable lifestyle, including his self-destructive behavior, was experienced, at some deep level, as an expression of loyalty, and as a way of maintaining ties to his own background and the early world of his origin. For this young man, to live differently was to abandon his past.

In short, according to Fairbairn's object relations theory, a powerful motive for repeating early relationship patterns is that they represent ways of maintaining ties to early objects. But the reasons for the tenacity of these ties is not limited to one's need for security, at least not in the sense highlighted by attachment theory. If I understand Fairbairn correctly, these ties constitute one's very sense of self and the raw material of one's inner world. To be without them is to risk the loss of one's sense of self and the schizoid experience of an empty inner world.

Weiss and Sampson's (1986) emphasis on guilt as the primary factor that perpetuates "unconscious pathogenic beliefs" and early object ties is similar, in certain respects, to Fairbairn's emphasis on "devotion" and "obstinate attachment." That is, according to Weiss and Sampson unconscious pathogenic beliefs are most often sustained by fear that one's actions or aims will threaten one's relationship with parental figures and/or will harm them in some way. An example of such a pathogenic belief is the fear that separation from parents or pursuing one's ambitions will be at their expense and/or harm them. It should also be noted that Freud, too, attempted to account for the rigid and persistent ties to early objects that one finds in certain individuals that he variously referred to as the "adhesiveness of the libido" (Freud, 1915a/1963, p. 272); "sluggishness of libidinal cathexis" (Freud, 1918/1955, p. 116); and "psychical inertia" (Freud, 1937a/1964, p. 242). But these, of course, are simply descriptions, in metapsychological language, of the phenomenon—and a surprisingly, nondynamic one—rather than an explanatory account.

ATTACHMENT THEORY AND RELATIONAL PSYCHOANALYSIS

One would think that there are natural affinities between attachment theory and relational psychoanalysis insofar as at the center of both perspectives is a primary emphasis on interpersonal interactions and their representations. And, indeed, there are such affinities. For example, Mitchell's (1988, p. 255) view of mind in terms of "transactional patterns" bears a strong family resemblance to Bowlby's (1973) concept of internal working model. Also, both Mitchell—the seminal theorist of relational psychoanalysis—and Bowlby reject Freudian drive theory and its corresponding concept of mind as a discharge apparatus.

However, there are also divergences that have mainly to do with differences in broad philosophical perspectives. For example, Mitchell (2002) does not appear to accept the legitimacy of an inborn instinctual attachment system and of the pursuit of security as an essential motive. In his book *Can Love Last?* he writes that the search for security "degrades" romance and is an illusory search. He also writes that "secure attachment" is not a terribly useful model of mutual, adult romantic love, except in its fantasy, illusory, security-bolstering dimensions. Love, by its very nature, is *not* secure; we keep wanting to make it so (p. 49). Mitchell seems to equate adult romantic love entirely as being at odds with the need for security.

One source of confusion here is that Mitchell equates love with sexual passion. When love is defined that way, it may, indeed, be partly incompatible with the search for security (see Chapter 8). However, long-term adult love relationships consist of a good deal more than sexual passion. And surely, safety and security are important and nonillusory aspects of these relationships. A more accurate title for Mitchell's book would be not *Can Love Last?*, but rather *Can Sexual Passion Last?*

Mitchell's views of mind and self are diametrically opposed to the positing of relatively stable structures such as internal working models. It also appears to be opposed to Mitchell's (1988) own earlier view of mind as comprising relatively stable "relational configurations." According to Mitchell (1998, 2000), whereas mind is "preexisting," it is not "preorganized." Rather, it is fluidly organized by ever-shifting interactions with others. He rejects the "traditional claims ... that the central dynamics relevant to the analytic process are pre-organized in the patient's mind" (p. 18). He also rejects the notion of a stable self structure and replaces it with the idea of multiple selves as a function of ongoing interpersonal interactions.

The concept of fluid multiple selves and self states (Bromberg, 1996) that fluctuate with each ongoing interaction is quite different from the idea of multiple internal working models that vary as a function of different attachment figures (e.g., mother vs. father). According to attachment theory, each working model is a relatively stable structure that is associated with an identified attachment figure rather than a fluid self state that fluctuates with each interaction.

Another point of divergence between attachment theory and relational psychoanalysis is reflected in Mitchell's (1998) dismissive attitude toward empirical research. As noted, at one point, he refers to the "Grunbaum syndrome," which is satirically characterized by "several days of guilty anguish for not having involved oneself in analytic research" and "may include actually trying to remember how analysis of variance works" as well as a "sleep disturbance and distractions from work." "However [he assures his readers], it invariably passes in a day or so, and the patient is able to return to a fully productive life" (p. 5).

The attitudes expressed in Mitchell's description of the "Grunbaum syndrome," I strongly suspect, are, as noted earlier, representative of the attitude of many analysts. In this regard, the divergence between the philosophical attitudes of many contemporary psychoanalysts and attachment theorists and researchers is perhaps almost as wide today as it was in Bowlby's day. In some respects, it may even be wider. I am referring to the explicit endorsement and adoption of an antiscientific perspective as well as of a postmodern philosophical attitude—which would have been anathema to Freud—on the part of at least some contemporary psychoanalytic theorists (see Eagle, 2003). One needs to note, however, that countering this trend is the emergence of an active and productive group of analytically oriented researchers and theorists (described by Fonagy, 2001) whose work reflects a healthy regard for empirical research as well as an increasing convergence of attachment theory and psychoanalytic perspectives.

ATTACHMENT THEORY AND SEPARATION–INDIVIDUATION

To a certain extent, although very different language is employed, Mahler's (1968; Mahler, Bergman, & Pine, 1975) formulation of the relationship between symbiosis and separation–individuation parallels the relationship between a secure base and exploration in attachment theory. However, Gullestad (2001) argues that little in attachment theory speaks directly to the child's need for separation and individuation, concepts that do not seem to entirely overlap with exploration. He observes that whereas Bowlby emphasizes separation in terms of the unavailability of the attachment figure, Mahler has in mind the child's need to achieve *psychological separation*, which is facilitated by the development of object constancy (which can be understood as the intrapsychic aspect of a secure base).

CHAPTER 7

Attachment and Infantile Sexuality

IS ATTACHMENT BASED ON PLEASURES ASSOCIATED WITH INFANTILE SEXUALITY?

In previous chapters, we have seen that secondary drive theory, which posits hunger reduction as the primary basis for infant–mother attachment, does not work. The choice of the hunger drive as a basis for a psychoanalytic account of infant–mother attachment always seemed an odd one insofar as it is infantile sexuality (e.g., oral gratification), not hunger, that is distinctly psychoanalytic. The seemingly odd choice of hunger lies, I believe, in the ease with which hunger reduction fits a biologically based tension–reduction–discharge model. Hunger and hunger satisfaction conform to a conception of drive characterized by the cyclical buildup and reduction or discharge of tension through a consummatory act. The parallel to Freud's conception of the sexual drive is apparent.

A far more distinctively psychoanalytic account is the claim that infant–mother attachment is based on infantile sexuality, that is, on the sensual pleasures associated with the erogenous zones stimulated in the course of the caregiver's ministrations of the infant. In commenting on Bowlby's (1960) paper, Anna Freud (1960) writes that "the infant has an inborn readiness to cathect with libido a person who provides pleasurable experiences" (p. 55). In this statement, Anna Freud does not distinguish between pleasurable experiences due to hunger reduction and those attendant upon stimulation of the erogenous zones. However, as noted, it is the latter that is distinctively psychoanalytic. For example, although sucking may originally be anaclitic upon the hunger drive, it is a more patent expression of infantile sexuality than hunger reduction. As Freud (1940/1964) puts it, "The baby's obstinate persistence in sucking gives evidence at an early stage of a need for satisfaction which, though it originates from and is integrated by the taking of nourishment, nevertheless strives to obtain pleasure independent of nourishment and for that reason may and should be termed sexual" (p. 154). Freud's own conception of infantile sexuality does not fit a tension or drive-reduction-discharge model. If the hallmark of infantile sexuality is sensual pleasure from stimulation of erogenous zones, then hunger and hunger satisfaction are poor representations of it.

In effect, Freud has two theories of pleasure: a quantitative one based on a drive or excitation-reduction model (ultimately resting on the constancy principle) and a qualitative one, the model of which is the kind of sensual pleasure linked to infantile sexuality and not easily conceptualized in tension reduction terms (see Klein, 1976, and Gillick & Bone, 1990). With regard to the latter, Freud (1924/1961) referred to certain forms of pleasure that "depend not on [a] quantitative factor, but on some characteristic of it which we can only describe as a qualitative one" (p. 160). Freud never adequately resolved the dilemma inherent in the recognition that there were qualitative aspects of pleasure that do not fit and even appear to be incongruent with his metapsychological quantitative conception of pleasure in terms of excitation reduction. He wrote with regard to the "qualitative factor" that "If we were able to say what this qualitative characteristic is, we should be much further advanced in psychology" (p. 160).

So, when in response to a paper by Bowlby (1960), Anna Freud (1960) states that the infant has an "inborn readiness to cathect with libido a person who provides pleasurable experiences" (p. 55), it is not clear how "pleasurable experiences" are understood. If, as some of her previous writings suggest, she has in mind the "pleasurable experiences" associated with hunger drive reduction, then Harlow's (1958) findings and attachment theory and research constitute a challenge to that view. If, on the other hand, she is referring to the sensual pleasures associated with sucking and tactile stimulation, then one could perhaps argue that her claim is not contradicted by, and perhaps is even congruent with, Harlow's findings insofar as the "contact comfort" identified by Harlow can be understood as a form of sensual pleasure.

Imagine that instead of invoking satisfaction of hunger, Freud simply argued that the infant becomes attached to mother because of the sensual pleasures she provides. (One is reminded here of Klein's [1976] suggestion that Freud's concept of infantile sexuality is best understood as *infantile sensuality*.) It would not be much of a stretch to say that that position is congruent with Harlow's (1958) claim that "contact comfort" is a critical basis for the infant monkey's attachment to its surrogate mother insofar as "contact comfort" suggests, among other things, pleasure associated with tactile stimulation. (Recall Freud's [1905/1953] idea that the entire surface of the infant's skin is an erogenous zone that yields pleasure when stimulated.)

Looked at from this perspective, one could argue that Harlow's findings provide support for Anna Freud's (1960) claim that the "infant has an inborn readiness to become attached to a person who provides pleasurable experiences" (p. 55)—recognizing that the "pleasurable experiences" associated with hunger reduction are not among those that rank high as a basis for infant–mother attachment. One could argue further that once one drops the emphasis on hunger drive reduction, there is no contradiction between Anna Freud's position and attachment theory insofar as Anna Freud acknowledges an inborn readiness to become attached—a central claim of attachment theory. One might say that whereas attachment theory formulates the evolutionary context of our inborn readiness to become attached, Anna Freud (as well as Harlow) points to the factors involved *in becoming attached to a specific person or object.*

What this rapprochement sloughs over, however, are those elements of traditional psychoanalytic theory that reject the idea of an inborn readiness to become attached to an object, elements that Anna Freud appears to ignore. Consider, for example, Freud's (1915b/1963) claim that the infant's earliest response to the object is one of "repulsion" and "hatred"—a claim based on the idea that the object disrupts the infant's supposed state of nirvana. Also, Freud (1900) argues that the reality of the object is something the infant only reluctantly confronts mainly because it is necessary for drive gratification or drive reduction. According to the logic of Freud's theorizing, were the infant to live in a world in which mere wishing would make it so, he or she would never develop an interest in objects or attachment to objects—that is, would never develop object relations. This view is hardly compatible with the assumptions of an inborn readiness to become attached and is diametrically opposed to the basic assumptions of attachment theory (as well as to Fairbairn's [1952] object relations theory).

In short, when Anna Freud (1960) acknowledges an inborn readiness to become attached, she does not also acknowledge that this is a major shift in the traditional psychoanalytic theory of psychological development and of human nature. Nor does she address the implications of acknowledging an inborn readiness to become attached for other aspects of psychoanalytic theorizing, including the positing of an early stage of primary narcissism, the separation of the drive and the object, hallucinatory wish fulfillment, the quantitative conception of pleasure, the autoerotic nature of infantile sexuality, and so on. These central concepts and assumptions of traditional psychoanalytic theory are simply not compatible with the positing of an inborn readiness to become attached to the object. The acknowledgment of an inborn readiness to become attached requires the systematic modification of these assumptions, the result of which would be a very different psychoanalytic theory.

If this partial rapprochement between traditional psychoanalysis and attachment theory represented by Anna Freud's acknowledgment of an inborn readiness to become attached is to be convincing, one must also address another issue. It is not clear from an attachment theory perspective whether one would place pleasures of any kind—the pleasure of tension (hunger) reduction or the sensual pleasures of infantile sexuality—as the primary and necessary determinants of the particular figure to whom the infant becomes attached. From the perspective of attachment theory, the infant's attachment to caregiver is primarily based, not on the sensual pleasures (including those linked to tactile stimulation), but on (1) prolonged propinquity and (2) the infant's experience of *security and safety*. Although safety and security constitute experiences of well-being, they do not easily fit a model of pleasure, particularly concepts of pleasure that are embedded in libido theory. Of course, a fascinating question which, as far as I know, has not been systematically addressed, is why sensual stimuli such as tactile stimulation ("contact comfort") rather than hunger reduction should be especially conducive to the infant's experience of security and safety. That is, why should tactile stimulation be especially instrumental in the formation of an attachment bond? From an evolutionary perspective there are undoubtedly good adaptive reasons that this should be the case.

PUNISHMENT INTENSIFIES ATTACHMENT BEHAVIOR

Another problem with Anna Freud's account is that there is a good deal of evidence that the attachment bond does *not* depend on pleasurable experiences with the caregivers and does not follow a simple reward–punishment model. Indeed, it has been found in animal studies that *punishment strengthens rather than weakens the infant's attachment to its caregiver.* Even when mother is rigged up to emit a noxious stimulus such as a puff of air when her infant approaches her, the infant clings even more tightly to mother (Harlow, 1960). Thus, punishment resulted in an *intensification* rather than a weakening of the infantile attachment responses (e.g., clinging to mother). From the point of view of attachment theory, this outcome

is not difficult to understand. We know that distress activates the attachment system. In this case, just as the theory predicts, the distress generated
by the puff of air intensifies the infant's attachment behavior. Of course,
the source of distress is the mother, the very figure the infant turns to for
security in times of distress. But what is the infant to do? The very figure
who is emitting the noxious stimulus is the only game in town. There is no
one else to whom the infant can turn for security during distress. (It would
be interesting to determine what the infant would do if multiple attachment
figures were available. As far as I know, this study has not been done.)

For a wide range of situations, when animals and humans experience
pain, they learn to avoid the situation associated with the painful situation.
However, this does not appear to be the case with regard to attachment
behavior. There is evidence that rat pups are attracted to a pain-associated
odor if mother was present during learning (Moriceau & Sullivan, 2006).
There is also evidence that when mother is present during a painful event
experienced by rat pups, the usual amygdala activation is suppressed and
the stress hormone corticosterone is not released (Barr et al., 2009; Sullivan, Landers, Yeaman, & Wilson, 2000). As Sullivan and Lasly (2010)
note, "when the parent and the nest are themselves sources of danger, the
suppression of fear circuits in the amygdala still works" (p. 3). As they
also suggest, early in life, the survival imperative of forming an attachment bond appears to take priority over other forms of learning, such as
learning to avoid painful situations. In short, the infant's attachment to the
caregiver does not appear to depend on pleasurable experiences or to be a
function of a reward–punishment process.

The finding in animal studies that punishment intensifies attachment
response is congruent with clinical observations that children who are
neglected and abused continue their intense attachment to, and even idealization, of the very parental figure who has neglected and abused them.
More light is shed on this phenomenon by Fairbairn's (1952) object relations theory than by the traditional assumption that attachment is linked to
pleasurable experiences. As Fairbairn observes, mistreated children often
remain attached to their parent in the hope that if only they become worthy
enough, they will be loved. One must also keep in mind the consideration
that even an abusive caregiver has provided some degree of regulation and
associated feelings of well-being, as attested to by the infant's survival.

In short, contrary to Anna Freud's (1960) assertion, the formation of
an attachment bond between infant (or child) and caregiver does not appear
to depend, in any simple way, on the latter being the source of pleasurable
experiences. Although perhaps the infant and child's *pattern* of attachment
will vary with the degree to which the caregiver has provided pleasurable

or unpleasurable experiences, it is unlikely that this factor alone will determine either the *fact* of attachment or the particular figure to whom the infant becomes attached. One should not underestimate the role of sheer prolonged propinquity and physical presence as primary factors in determining to whom the infant becomes attached.

ATTACHMENT AND "CONTACT COMFORT"

I want to turn now to the question of why the experience of security should be specifically linked to "contact comfort," that is, to a particular *texture of the attachment figure* and the accompanying tactile stimulation that figure provides. Why was it not linked to the intake of milk in Harlow's (1958) study? One can speculate that if proximity to the caregiver is the "set goal" of the attachment system, then it makes good evolutionary sense that "contact comfort," which cannot be experienced without physical proximity, would be associated with feelings of security and would serve as a primary basis for the formation of an attachment bond. Just as sucking is anaclitic upon the biological necessity of feeding, so "contact comfort" may be anaclitic upon the biological necessity of proximity to the caregiver.

The factors and experiences that serve as critical bases for the infant's attachment to its caregiver cannot be determined a priori and are likely to vary with the particular species studied. Thus, whereas for monkeys, "contact comfort" seems to be a central basis for attachment, for rat pups olfactory stimulation appears to be critical. Thus, as Hofer (1990) has shown, if, after the first few days of life, rat pups are deprived of their olfactory sense, "they show no apparent interest in their mother, treating her like an inanimate object. They ultimately die of inanition despite her continued presence with them" (pp. 63–64). It appears, then, that without an intact olfactory sense, rat infants would not be capable of becoming attached despite an inborn readiness to becoming attached. This is obviously not the case in other species where olfaction does not play as central a role as it does for rats. However, olfactory stimulation appears to interact with tactile and other stimulation in contributing to the mammalian development of attachment to the caregiver. As Hofer (1990) notes, "infant mammals are highly adapted to finding their way about the ventrum of their mothers, an environment filled with soft tactile, thermal, and olfactory stimulation" (p. 62).

The identification of the specific factors that are implicated in the infant's attachment to its caregiver reveals, by contrast, the relative vacuousness of general theories that refer only to such abstract and vague concepts as drive or tension reduction or person who provides pleasurable experiences.

As we have seen in Chapter 3, the mother's stimulus "inputs" regulate a wide range of physiological and behavioral systems in the infant. Such regulation is likely to be accompanied by feelings of well-being and some forms of pleasure; and the withdrawal of these "inputs" that lead to dysregulation of the infant are likely to be accompanied by feelings of distress and unpleasure. Hofer has suggested that an addiction model captures the nature of the infant's early attachment to mother. That is, the stimulation and "substances" provided by mother produce feelings of well-being, and their withdrawal produces feelings of distress. In this sense, the infant becomes "addicted" to the mother's regulatory provisions. Hofer (1990) also speculates "that the presence of multiple independent processes of altered regulatory control during separation may supply, at the biological level, a basis for the quality of fragmentation and loss of control that characterizes the experience of object loss and the affects of grief in humans" (p. 70). One can understand the above findings as elucidating some of the specific physiological processes that serve as a foundation for the infant's later psychological attachment to its caregiver.

This is as it should be. For it is the function of empirical research to sharpen and make more precise such general terms as "pleasurable experiences." As an example of this process, consider Spitz's (1965) concept of "auxiliary ego" and his findings on the dire effects of the lack of a consistent caregiver on the infant's development. With regard to the former, in the light of subsequent research, the concept of "auxiliary ego" can now be "filled in" and understood in the context of the specific early regulatory functions of the caregiver; with regard to the latter, Spitz's account of the marasmus, which makes reference to such vague formulations as the absence of objects on to which the infant can discharge sexual and aggressive tensions, can now be replaced with an account that identifies the specific regulatory functions of which the infant is deprived and the specific consequences of their unavailability.

What remains to be dealt with are the findings indicating that punishment at the hands of the caregiver intensifies the infant's attachment behavior. Do not the findings contradict the idea that experiences of wellbeing linked to the regulatory function of the caregiver form an early basis for attachment to a specific figure? Indeed, they do not. For the findings reported by Hofer and others speak to the early basis of the specific figure to whom the infant becomes attached, whereas the findings on effects of punishment have to do with the intensified activation of attachment behavior in the context of an existing attachment bond. *They do not pertain to the basis for the attachment that is formed.* Even a neglectful and abusive caregiver has provided not only prolonged propinquity, but also some degree of the kind of physiological regulation described by Hofer. If that were not the case, the infant would not survive. So, the point is that even with neglectful and abusive caregivers, the preconditions for attachment are present. If the neglect and abuse are too extreme, either the infant does not survive or if he or she does, there is a greatly increased risk that the attachment system is compromised, as reflected in either failure to develop an attachment bond or indiscriminate attachment—two sides of the same coin (Zeanah et al., 2005).

THE AUTOEROTIC NATURE OF INFANTILE SEXUALITY

Still another problem with the proposal that the pleasures associated with infantile sexuality serve as the primary basis for attachment to a specific figure is the identification of infantile sexuality with autoerotic pleasures and fantasies in Freudian theory. We are told by Freud (1905/1953) (as well as other psychoanalytic theorists, for example, Widlocher, 2002) that the hallmark of infantile sexuality is its *autoerotic* nature. As Freud writes, infantile sexuality "has as yet no sexual object, and is thus auto-erotic" (p. 182). And by autoerotic he means that the infant "finds its object in the infant's own body" (p. 197). (Freud refers to thumb-sucking and masturbation as prime examples of the autoerotic nature of infantile sexuality.) It is only at the onset of puberty, Freud tells us, that "the sexual instinct [which] has hitherto been predominantly auto-erotic ... now finds a sexual object" (p. 207).

　　The obvious question is: If infantile sexuality is inherently autoerotic and independent of the object, how can it, at the same time, constitute the primary basis for the infant's attachment to mother? In order for infantile sexuality to be relevant to attachment, the infant must make some connection between the pleasures experienced and the person who provides them. Thus, the fundamental autoerotic nature of infantile sexuality posited by Freud seems to utterly contradict Anna Freud's (1960) formulation that the infant becomes attached to "a person who provides pleasurable experiences" (p. 55).

　　Freud (1925a/1959) does write that "after the stage of auto-eroticism, the first love object in the case of both sexes is the mother" (p. 36). But what is not clear is (1) why a stage of autoeroticism is assumed in the first place and (2) how long this supposed stage lasts. In *Three Essays on the Theory of Sexuality*, Freud (1905/1953) clearly implies that it lasts until the onset of puberty. He writes, in regard to puberty, that "the sexual instinct has hitherto been predominantly auto-erotic; it now finds a sexual object" (p. 207). This formulation seems to contradict the claim that "after the stage of auto-eroticism, the first love object for both sexes is the mother." Also, does the mother become the first love object for both sexes at puberty? Surely not. Also, in the light of Freud's formulation of the Oedipus complex, which entails the cathexis of a sexual object outside of the child's own body, what does it mean to say that only at the onset of puberty does the sexual instinct find a sexual object? In short, the entire set of theoretical formulations regarding infantile sexuality, autoeroticism, and attachment is confused and confusing.

In the book *Infantile Sexuality and Attachment*, Widlocher (2002) follows through on what seems to be a logical implication of Freud's views on infantile sexuality. Pushing these views to their logical conclusion, as well as taking account of other views, such as Balint's concept of primary love and Bowlby's attachment theory, Widlocher severs any connection between infantile sexuality and attachment. He distinguishes sharply between, on the one side, the autoerotic nature of pleasure-seeking which is characterized by fantasy (internal psychic activity), autoerotic activity, and the interchangeability of objects, and on the other side, object-love and attachment, which involves a specific and real object in the world.

For Widlocher, "infantile sexuality takes form as a result of an internal demand and achieves satisfaction in psychic and/or autoerotic activity" (p. 13). This psychic activity, Widlocher tells us, is entirely in the realm of fantasy and imagination. Most important in the present context, according to Widlocher, infantile sexuality has little or nothing to do with the development of attachment. Unlike the fantasy-saturated nature of infantile sexuality, Widlocher notes, attachment is linked to the real world and to ties to real objects in that world.

When Widlocher severs the link between infantile sexuality and attachment, he is, I believe, accurately spelling out the implications of Freud's position. As Widlocher puts it, "[The object] is only the actor called upon to play a role in the imaginary scenario. It is interchangeable, and the same object can play different parts in the same scenario. Wish fulfillment ... is the goal that is sought and the source of pleasure" (p. 13). Here, Widlocher is being true to Freud's conception of the autoerotic nature of infantile sexuality and the relatively peripheral and interchangeable role played by the object. For Widlocher, as for Freud, the autoerotic nature of infantile sexuality expresses "the more general hedonic tendency to produce pleasure by hallucinating satisfaction" (p. 22).

Put another way, for Widlocher, infantile sexuality "expresses an imaginary relation to the object" (p. 21), whereas object-seeking and object love are directed toward real objects in the world. According to Widlocher, psychic life is characterized by a constant and "conflictual interweaving of love for the other and the quest for autoerotic pleasure" (p. 31).

In ceding that object-seeking (Fairbairn), primary object love (Balint), and an inborn attachment system (Bowlby) are the basis for the establishment of infant–mother attachment, Widlocher and the other contributors to the volume *Infantile Sexuality and Attachment* are relinquishing Freud's and Anna Freud's claim that it is infantile sexuality that is the basis for infant–mother attachment. They are, in effect, acknowledging two separate systems, one linked to infant–mother attachment and other, infantile sexuality, characterized by pleasure-seeking, autoerotic activity, and fantasy. Freud (1915a/1963) himself, in some of his writings, suggests just such a distinction when he writes about the differences between the self-preservative and the sexual or libidinal instincts.

As noted in Chapter 8, in his 1912/1957 essay, where he focuses on the split between the "affectionate and sensual currents," Freud writes that "the affectionate current is the older of the two" and "corresponds to the child's primary object choice" (p. 180). Freud is suggesting here that the child's "primary object-choice," that is, his or her attachment bond to mother, is based on an autonomous self-preservative instinct independent of sexuality, although the sexual instincts then attach themselves to the object already "selected" by the self-preservative instinct—much like the way sexual-sensual pleasures of erogenous zones attach themselves to and are experienced in relation to bodily functions (e.g., feeding, elimination) and zones. As noted earlier, read in a particular way, one can understand Freud as virtually anticipating Bowlby's claim that the infant's attachment to mother is based on an independent (self-preservative) instinctual system (see Silverman, 1991).

However, Freud (1) relinquished his earlier dual instinct theory of self-preservative and libidinal instincts and replaced it with the dual sexual and aggressive instinct theory; (2) he also presented a secondary drive theory (based on hunger reduction and pleasures from erogenous zones) of infant–mother attachment, which is at odds with his "primary object-choice" theory and which was given priority by Anna Freud; and (3) he never made entirely clear how infantile sexuality is linked to "primary object-choice," nor did he present convincing evidence that they are closely linked. In a certain sense, one can partly understand Bowlby's work as filling out, elaborating, and modernizing Freud's earlier unelaborated views regarding the child's "primary object-choice" in the light of empirical findings as well as initiating a relevant research program.

It should be noted that for the mainly French contemporary Freudian analysts represented in the Widlocher volume, issues of attachment, security, and real events are of relatively little interest to psychoanalysis. For them, psychoanalysis is mainly concerned with the autoerotic fantasies of infantile sexuality and their persistence into adult psychic life.

For this reason, the suggestion on the jacket of the Widlocher volume that the book is concerned with the question of whether attachment rests on infantile sexuality or on an autonomous instinctual attachment system is misleading. Rather, most of the contributors to the volume are not especially interested in attachment and related matters. They cede that territory to those who study the "real" or "natural" or "observed" child (Green, 2000). Furthermore, unlike Freud and Anna Freud, they do not push the claim that infant–mother attachment is based on infantile sexuality, which they discuss as quite independent of the formation of actual infant–mother attachment. Their interest is in the "true" child of psychoanalysis, the child of infantile sexuality, of autoerotic activity, and of fantasy.

It turns out that what Green (2000), Widlocher (2002), and the contributors to the Widlocher volume mean by the "true" child of psychoanalysis is the child as inferentially constructed from the production of adult psychoanalytic patients. Green, Widlocher, and the others have no interest in data from infant observations or the "real" child of developmental psychology. Their interest is in what they believe to be the active residues of infantile sexuality—its autoerotic fantasies—in adult mental life. For them, the task of psychoanalysis is to identify these residues, including their relationship to one's capacity for love of the actual other—as Widlocher puts it, "the conflictual interweaving of love for the other and the quest for auto-erotic pleasure" (p. 31).

Thus, Widlocher (2002) is essentially proposing that at least infantile sexuality (or more accurately, the residues of infantile sexuality in adult mental life) and attachment, while interacting with each other, are distinct and functionally separable systems. It is this issue that is taken up in the next chapter.

CHAPTER 8

Attachment and Adult Sexuality[1]

Any discussion of attachment and psychoanalytic theories needs to include a consideration of the relationship between attachment and sexuality, given the central role sexuality plays in classical psychoanalytic theory. Until recently there has been a paucity of literature on the topic. Bowlby's focus (and that of his coworkers and followers) was on presenting a systematic and compelling case for the existence of an autonomous instinctual attachment system and on developing attachment theory. The explosion of research and theory that followed Bowlby's work focused on the complexities and details of the attachment system and had little to say about sexuality or the relationship between sexuality and attachment.

With the autonomy of the attachment system pretty much established, attention could turn to exploration of the relationship between that system and sexuality. Such an exploration is also facilitated by two additional factors: (1) the extension of attachment research to *adult attachment* in which it is one's romantic or sexual partner who is most frequently defined as one's attachment figure and (2) the recognition that, although closely related, the attachment and sexual systems are separable.

---

[1]This chapter is based on Eagle (2007).

ATTACHMENT AND SEXUALITY AS FUNCTIONALLY SEPARABLE SYSTEMS

Although Bowlby focused mainly on attachment, he did make a number of comments about the relationship between attachment and sexuality. He observed that in contrast to Freudian theory, which essentially viewed attachment as a product of (infantile) sexuality, according to attachment theory, the attachment and sexual behavioral systems are distinct systems. As Bowlby (1969/1982) noted, "the activation of the two systems vary independently of each other" and "the class of objects toward which each is directed may be quite different" (p. 231). However, "although regarded as distinct behavioral systems, attachment behavior and sexual behavior are believed to have unusually close linkages" (p. 230).

Although they interact with each other, Bowlby is correct in suggesting that attachment and sexuality are distinctive and separable behavioral systems. Holmes (2001) has commented that it is not uncommon to observe intense attachment without sexual interest and intense sexual interest without attachment. Fonagy (2001) makes a similar observation in noting that "the facts that sex can undoubtedly occur without attachment and that marriages without sex perhaps represent the majority of such partnerships, prove beyond a doubt that these systems are separate and at most loosely coupled" (p. 10).

There is a good deal of evidence supporting this conclusion: For example, in a recent study on factors that contribute to the experience of intimacy and romantic relationships, attachment to partner made the greatest contribution followed by sensitivity to caregiving. The authors note that "a surprising finding was that measures of sexual behavior ... did not make a unique contribution to intimacy in romantic relationships" (Farrugia & Hogans, 1998, p. 11). This finding is especially noteworthy given the young age of the sample. It should be noted, however, that the sample was predominantly female and that the authors did not report results for males and females separately. Nevertheless, the results tend to support the conclusion of Waring, Tillman, Frelick, Russell, and Weisz (1980) "that sexuality is considered part of intimacy by most people, although it is not considered to be the primary component" (p. 4).

Taking an evolutionary perspective, Diamond (2003) argues that "the evolved processes underlying sexual desire and affectional bonding are functionally independent" and that "although sexual desire and romantic love are often experienced in concert, they are governed by different social-behavioral systems that evolved to serve different goals" (p. 174). As Diamond notes, and as noted earlier in my citation of Holmes's (2001) and Fonagy's (2001) observations, one expression of the functional independence of the attachment and sexual systems is the fact that humans can bond without experiencing sexual desire and can experience sexual desire without bonding. According to Diamond (see also Fisher, 1998), "desire is governed by the *sexual mating* system" (p. 174), the goal of which is reproduction, whereas romantic love[2] is governed by the attachment or pair-bonding system ... the goal of which is the maintenance of an enduring association" (p. 174) for the purpose of survival of dependent offspring. Diamond presents the intriguing and likely to be correct idea that pair-bonding or attachment originally evolved, not in the context of sexual mating but instead "exploited" the already existing infant–caregiver attachment system "for the purpose of maintaining enduring associations between adult reproductive partners" (p. 174). In other words, it is primarily attachment, not sex, that keeps adult partners together for a long period of time.

Biological Evidence

There is intriguing evidence that the attachment and sexual systems are mediated by different biological processes. As Liebowitz (1983) observes: "Biologically, it appears that we have evolved two distinct chemical systems for romance; one basically serves to bring people together and the other to keep them together. The first is [sexual] attraction ... the second, which helps keep people together, is attachment. Attachment has more to do with feelings of security than of excitement" (p. 90). There is evidence that the sexual attraction phase of a relationship is accompanied by a higher level of amphetamine-like substances, especially phenyethylanine, which is associated with heightened arousal and activity, whereas the attachment phase is accompanied by endorphin release, which is also associated with the formation of infant–mother affectional bonds.

There is much evidence that oxytocin and vasopressin play an important role in both maternal behavior and mother–infant bonding. Oxytocin facilitates the onset of maternal behavior in rats and facilitates the acceptance of an alien lamb in a nonpregnant ewe. Prairie voles, which are monogamous, have different distributions of oxytocin and vasopressin receptors in the brain from montane voles, which are nonmonogamous.

---

[2]I am not at all sure that "romantic love" is the best term to describe adult attachment. For, as Mitchell (2002) has noted, there is often very little romance remaining in long-term adult attachments. Perhaps the more neutral terms "adult attachment" or "pair-bonding" are more accurate.

As Insel and Young (2001) note, "vasopressin receptors in the ventral pallidum are present not only in prairie voles but also in monogamous mice and primates whereas they are absent in this region in related rodent and primate species that do not form pair bonds" (p. 133). They also note, "all the major aspects of monogamy can be facilitated in the prairie vole by central injection of either oxytocin or vasopressin, even in montane voles that do not have the opportunity to mate" (pp. 132–133). Furthermore, when an oxytocin receptor antagonist is injected into the female prairie vole, the usual monogamous preference for a partner is blocked. All this and other evidence tend to support Diamond's (2003) reasoning that "if the biobehavioral process underlying romantic love [Diamond is clearly referring to an attachment bond here] originally evolved in the context of infant caregiver attachment ... then the oxytocinergic mechanisms reviewed above should also underlie adult pair-bonding" (p. 181). During the last few years, some fascinating findings have emerged on the relationship between oxytocin and a number of behaviors that are linked to attachment. For example, intranasal oxytocin (along with social support) lowers cortisol release during stress (Heinrichs, Baumgartner, Kirschbaum, & Ehlert, 2003) and also enhances secure attachment as measured by the AAI (Buchheim et al., 2009). Consistent with these findings, a higher level of oxytocin is associated with greater trust (Zak, Kurzban, & Matzner, 2005). Adult attachment classification also predicts maternal brain and oxytocin response to infant cues (Strathearn, Fonagy, Amico, & Montague, 2009).

In seeming incongruence with the aforementioned findings, Marazziti et al. (2006) reported a positive relationship between attachment anxiety on the ECR and level of oxytocin. However, they interpret their findings as indicating that oxytocin is released in order to deal with anxiety. In accord with this interpretation, Tops, Van Peer, Korf, Wijers, and Tucker (2007) found that stress induces oxytocin release which, in the context of support, relieves stress. The role of oxytocin in relieving stress is also suggested by the findings that when oxytocin release is deactivated, adrenocorticotropic hormone secretion is released.

As another example of physiological contributions to the disjunction between attachment and sexuality, middle-aged men and women who were administered testosterone to increase sexual desire reported experiencing increased sexual thoughts and elevated levels of sexual activity, but did not report feeling increased romantic passion or increased attachment to their partners (Fisher, 2000, p. 415; Sherwin & Gelfand, 1987; Sherwin, Gelfand, & Brender, 1985).

PARTIAL ANTAGONISM BETWEEN ATTACHMENT AND SEXUALITY

Physiological Evidence

There is a good deal of evidence in both animals and humans indicating the effects of testosterone on monogamous and polygamous behavior. For example, with regard to the former, Wingfield (1984) reported that subcutaneous implantation of testosterone in monogamous birds renders them polygamous.

A similar effect of testosterone in humans is shown in a variety of ways: For example, single men and women have higher levels of testosterone than partnered men and women. However, partnered men who reported greater desire for uncommitted sex had the same level of testosterone as single men. And partnered women who reported more frequent uncommitted sexual behavior had the same level of testosterone as single women (Edelstein, Chopik, & Kean, 2011).

In a study of 890 men, Kuzawa, Gettler, Muller, McDade, and Feranil (2009) found that young fathers had a lower level of testosterone than single men. In another study, Kuzawa, Gettler, Huang, and McDade (2010) reported that young mothers and partnered women had lower waking testosterone than single women. This was particularly true of mothers of young infants. Furthermore, these findings were independent of breastfeeding, contraceptive pill use, sleep quality, menstrual cycle, employment, and socioeconomic status.

In a rather striking finding, Gettler, Agustin, McDade, and Kuzawa (2011) reported that although there was no change in testosterone level, levels of cortisol and prolactin declined minutes after men played with their children. And finally, in a study of more than 700 elderly men and women, Pollett et al. (2011) found that testosterone level was associated with number of lifetime sex partners reported by men even after controlling for possible confounding variables such as age, level of education, and ethnicity. A similar but weaker relationship was found for women.

Freud's View

Freud (1912/1957), commented not only on the separability between "love and desire" and the "affectionate and sensual currents"—which, it is clear from the context, are roughly equivalent to attachment and sexuality (more on that later)—but also on the conflictual relationship between the two. He characterized a group of men suffering from "psychical impotence" in the following way: "where they love they do not desire and where they desire they cannot love" (p. 183). He also made clear his belief that even if not expressed in the symptomatic form of psychical impotence, the split between love and desire was quite common in both men and women and took the form of lack of sexual enjoyment and interest in relation to one's spouse or long-term partner.[3]

How does one account for this seeming disjunction and conflict between the attachment and sexual behavioral systems? Freud's response to the question is quite clear: The individual's inability to combine the affectionate and sexual currents is due, Freud (1912/1957) writes, to "an incestuous fixation on mother or sister which has never been surmounted" (p. 180). Normally, the individual will find a way to "extraneous objects with which a real sexual life may be carried on" (p. 181). But this normal trajectory will be interfered with if there is a continuing excessive "attraction" (p. 181) of infantile (incestuous) objects. The continuing attraction of infantile objects means that the sexual feelings, the sexual act, and the anticipation of the sexual act will trigger unconscious incestuous fantasies which, of course are forbidden. The end result is the split between love and desire.

Freud notes that psychical impotence occurs with certain partners and not with others. Potency is possible only with "objects which do not recall the incestuous figures forbidden to it" (pp. 182–183), that is, with those who do not trigger the "affectionate current" and who are not held in "high psychical estimation." When "someone makes an impression that might lead to a high psychical estimation" (p. 183), one finds the absence of "sensual excitement," and instead "an affection which has no erotic effect" (p. 183).

As Freud (1912/1957) puts it, "they seek objects which do not lead to love in order to keep their sensuality away from objects they love" (p. 183). Further, even when "an object which has been chosen with the aim of avoiding incest [nevertheless] recalls the prohibited object," the result is impotence. More broadly, the result is the split between the affectionate and sensual currents: As noted, "where they love they do not desire and where they desire they cannot love" (p. 183). In short, for Freud the split between love and desire, and between the "affectionate and sensual currents," is characteristic of unresolved Oedipal conflicts and is mainly due to

---

[3] Although Freud includes women in his account of the split between love and desire, as his term "psychical impotence" and his reference to incestuous desires toward mother and sister indicate, his discussion is directed mainly to male sexuality. The question of whether his formulations regarding the split between love and desire are applicable to women is taken up later in the chapter.

the persistence of unconscious incestuous wishes and the need to keep such wishes diverted from objects one loves.[4]

One must remember that, according to Freud's account, incestuous wishes not only occur in early life, but *persist unconsciously with unabated intensity* into adulthood even after one has left one's family of origin. As we have seen, according to Freud, it is the persistence of these wishes into adulthood (combined with the persistence of the incest taboo) that accounts for the widespread split between love and desire. For Freud (1912/1957), so unrelenting are incestuous wishes that "anyone who is to be really free and happy in love must have ... come to terms with the idea of incest with his mother or sister" (p. 186). But the civilized man cannot do this. "There are only a few educated people," Freud tells us, "in whom the two currents of affection and sensuality have become properly fused" (p. 185). The best one can do, according to Freud, is to choose an "extraneous object" who will, however, "still be chosen on the model (imago) of the infantile ones" (p. 181). But the "realization of complete satisfaction" (p. 189) will be barred because "the final object of the sexual instinct is never any longer the original object but only a surrogate for it." The result is a continuous craving consequent upon always having to accept substitutes, never the original object.

This state of affairs, Freud makes clear, though more exaggerated and pronounced in neurosis, is in fact widespread and normative in the "civilized man" (p. 184). The clear implication of Freud's formulation is that were it not for the incest taboo, men, that is, adult men, not just children, would choose the path of unbridled and "complete satisfaction" inherent in the gratification of incestuous wishes, the path "to be really free and happy in love" (p. 186). The picture that emerges from Freud's writings is a psychological state of affairs in which early incestuous wishes based on one's original "love affair" with mother, persist throughout life and in combination with the incest taboo, influence the individual's capacity to combine feelings of sexual desire and love toward the same person.

Mitchell's View

Mitchell (2002) notes that the split between love and desire observed by Freud is as prevalent today as it was in Freud's day. However, according to Mitchell, the primary reason for the split between love and desire is not the

---

[4]In his 1912 essay in which, as the Editor notes, Freud uses the term "Oedipus complex" for the first time, he focuses exclusively on incestuous wishes. When he more fully develops the concept of the Oedipus complex, he also discusses the child's rivalrous wishes toward the opposite sex parent.

persistence of incestuous desires, but the motivation to "degrade romance." This is, he states, because one needs to render it secure, predictable, and safe, characteristics that, he maintains, are inimical to the experience of desire. According to Mitchell, in order to feel safe and secure, one needs to make the other familiar and predictable. However, he goes on, this very familiarity and predictability dulls romantic desire and sexual excitement. He argues that "it is not that romance itself has a tendency to become degraded, but that we expend considerable effort degrading it for good reasons" (p. 28). The good reasons Mitchell has in mind mainly have to do with the need to make love safe—"to establish security" (p. 44)—by making it more predictable. But by trying to make love safe, we are "thereby undermining the preconditions of desire, which require robust imagination to breathe and thrive" (p. 47).

Mitchell illustrates his formulation with case material in which the patient (Susan) needed to keep her marriage "dull and predictable" and reserve the excitement for a sexual affair. The dullness and predictability, according to Mitchell, is what keeps her marriage safe. He tells us that "when patients complain of dead and lifeless marriages, it is often possible to show them how precious the deadness is to them, how the very mechanical, totally predictable quality of lovemaking serves as a bulwark against the dread of surprise and unpredictability" (p. 49). Mitchell concludes his discussion of Susan by stating, "Thus, 'secure attachment' is not a terribly useful model of mutual, adult romantic love, except in its faulty, illusory, secure-bolstering dimensions. Love, by its very nature, is *not* secure; we keep wanting to make it so" (p. 49).

According to Mitchell, then, the split between sex and love, the fading and degradation of romance, is something we *need*, something we bring about in order to feel safe and more secure. Thus, while people may complain about the dullness and deadness of their relationship, that very dullness and deadness is "precious to them" because it protects them against the danger and dread of "surprise and unpredictability." He writes, "We become attached and we want objects of our attachment to stay fixed, unchanging. So ironically enough, attachment is the great enemy of eroticism" (p. 87).

Mitchell notes that "the precondition of romantic passion is lack, that desire for what one does not have" (p. 56). When one tries to remove that lack through security and commitment, Mitchell writes, the "allure is lost" (p. 56). Mitchell's linking of romantic passion with "lack, desire for what one does not have," parallels Lacan's (1960/2006) discussion of desire as well as Freud's (1912/1957) observation that "the psychical value of erotic needs is reduced as soon as their satisfaction becomes easy. An obstacle is required in order to heighten libido" (p. 187). However, unlike Freud, who believes that the diminution of erotic passion that accompanies easy satisfaction lies in the very nature of sexuality, Mitchell maintains that we are *motivated* to degrade passion; it is something we *seek* to accomplish or bring about.

Critique of Freud's View

As noted, according to Freud, the inability to combine love and desire is due to the persistence of incestuous wishes. The broader context of the claim are the linchpin assumptions, embodied in Freud's theory of infantile sexuality and of the Oedipus complex which posits that we all harbor powerful incestuous wishes and impulses, accompanied by an equally powerful incest taboo. For Freud, the split between love and desire is ultimately the product of the incest taboo operating in the face of a persistent incestuous fixation. Although individuals may differ in how they deal with incestuous wishes, according to Freud, these wishes are universal and powerful.

Although there is much evidence for a universal or at least near universal incest *taboo*, there is much controversy regarding the existence of powerful and universal incestuous *wishes*. Instead of providing direct evidence of universal incestuous wishes, the standard argument has been that the very presence of a powerful and universal cultural taboo is sufficient ground for inferring the existence of equally universal and powerful incestuous wishes that the taboo is intended to keep in check. This reasoning is illustrated very clearly, for example, by Lindzey (1967):

> One may argue persuasively that the mere universal existence of the incest taboo, together with the powerful effects of emotions that are associated with its violation, constitute convincing evidence for the existence of a set of general tendencies that are being denied. It seems unlikely that there would have been universal selection in favor of such a taboo if there were not rather widespread impulses toward expression of the prohibition. (p. 1055)

Essentially the same argument was stated by Freud (1916–1917) when he wrote that, "we should be at a loss to understand the necessity for stern prohibitions, which would seem to point to a strong desire" (p. 210).

It seems to me that the argument that there would be no "need" for a universal and strong taboo were there not powerful urges and impulses against which the taboo is enacted as a barrier is a faulty one—the near universal taboo against suicide or bestiality or murder or theft, for example, does not constitute adequate evidence that we have universal suicidal, bestial, murderous, or criminal wishes and urges that need to be held in check by the taboos and prohibitions against them. As Fox (1980) points out, "we need not assume that we have laws against murder because we all have murderous natures, but only because *some* murder occurs and we don't like that" (p. 8).

Similarly, one would say that we have an incest taboo not because we all have incestuous natures, but because the cost of even *some* incest is to be avoided. Fox observes that "there are many tribes and nations ... that do not effectively punish either, but that are not overwhelmed with incest or murder" (p. 7). He suggests that the proper question is not, "Why do human beings not commit incest?" but "Why do human beings not *want* [italics added] to commit incest all that much?" (p. 7). Fox goes on to observe with regard to incest that "*unease* and *avoidance* seem to be the common denominators—not fierce sanctions or lust reined in by the power of taboo" (p. 9).

Of course, Freud would counter that one finds unease and avoidance and not fierce *conscious* incestuous desire because such desire has been defended against and thus has become unconscious. Indeed, as Lindzey (1967) does, Freud would take the general unease and avoidance in response to incest as *betraying* unconscious incestuous desire. But this does not take one very far in responding to the challenge of presenting more direct evidence for the claim that powerful incestuous wishes and impulses—even if unconscious ones—are universal.

It is interesting to observe that the topic of incest originally entered psychoanalysis in the context, not of the child's incestuous wishes toward parents, but of *adult incestuous seduction of children.* When Freud rejected his seduction theory and replaced it with the theory of universal seduction *fantasies,* the direction was reversed and the focus was now on the child rather than the adult as the "carrier" of incestuous wishes and impulses. The fact is, however, that when the incest taboo is violated and incest occurs, it is initiated by the adult, not the child. So Freud's shift from actual seduction to seduction fantasy is not occasioned by new clinical/empirical evidence (see Israels & Schatzman, 1993). Rather, it is required by his theory of infantile sexuality and of the Oedipal complex.

The Westermarck Hypothesis

As early as 1891, Westermarck observed that, "generally speaking, there is a remarkable absence of erotic feelings between persons living very closely together from childhood. Nay, more, in this, as in many other cases, sexual indifference is combined with the positive feeling of aversion when the act is thought of" (Westermarck, 1926, p. 80). The absence of erotic feeling, even sexual aversion, in these circumstances, Westermarck proposes, serves to effect the avoidance of incest and the facilitation of exogamy. Freud was aware of the "Westermarck effect," but summarily dismissed it at various points. At one point, he writes, "If living together dampens sexual desire toward those with whom one grows up, an avoidance of incest would be secured automatically, and it would not be clear why such severe prohibitions were called for, which would point rather to the presence of a strong desire for it" (1916–1917/1961, p. 210). He also writes:

> It has been said that sexual inclination is diverted from members of the same family who are of the opposite sex by the fact of having been together from childhood. ... In all of this the fact is entirely overlooked that such an inexorable prohibition of it in law and custom would not be needed if there were any reliable natural barriers against the temptation of incest. The truth is just the opposite. A human being's first choice of an object is regularly an incestuous one, aimed in the case of the male, at his mother and sister. (pp. 334–335)

Apart from the earlier noted inadequacy of this argument, the idea that universal biologically based incestuous wishes are held in check by cultural restraints is entirely upended by the finding—of which Freud could not possibly be aware—that incest avoidance is present in a wide range of animal species. This finding suggests that we need to turn Freud's argument on its head. It is the incest taboo that is biologically based (the product of natural selection) and incestuous desires and actions that appear to be a cultural product.

There is also evidence that strongly suggests that, in accord with the Westermarck hypothesis, across a wide range of species, prolonged propinquity and familiarity dampen sexual interest, whereas unfamiliarity, novelty, and diversity intensify it. For example, as Fox (1980) notes, "Evidence exists from animals, moths, and birds that opposite-sex creatures reared together during immaturity copulate less readily than strangers when mature" (p. 24).[5]

In one study, Talmon (1964) looked at 125 marriages in three well-established kibbutzim and found not a single case in which two people reared in the same peer group had married. In a larger study, Shepher (1971)

---

[5] As will be seen later in this chapter, the story is somewhat more complicated. Although both animals and humans avoid sex with those with whom they were reared, they tend to show a greater preference for mates who are "optimally similar" to those with whom they were reared than for mates who are either totally unrelated or too closely related to those with whom they were reared. I discuss possible implications of this finding later in the chapter.

obtained the records of 2,769 marriages of people raised on kibbutzim. He found only 16 cases in which people reared together in the same group married. Furthermore, in all 16 of these apparent exceptions, not a single marriage occurred between people who had been reared together between birth and 6 years of age. Shepher notes that there were also publicly known love affairs, but his data in this area are more impressionistic than systematic. In accord with the Westermarck hypothesis, Shepher concludes that a "negative imprinting" with regard to incest is established during the first 6 years of life.

Shor and Simchai (2009) presented a critique of the Westermarck hypothesis and, in particular, of the Shepher study on the following grounds: (1) The Shepher study did not produce evidence of sexual aversion, but only of nonmarriage among kibbutzim peers; (2) the number of marriages is not a valid measure of sexual attraction; (3) the kibbutz peers were not asked about their sexual attraction to each other; and (4) Shepher did not take account of the role of group cohesion and prohibitions on the kibbutz in trying to account for the relative absence of love affairs and marriage among peers.

In an attempt to provide data on (3) and (4), Shor and Simchai conducted 60 in-depth interviews with individuals who grew up on kibbutzim. They reported that "almost none of the interviewees reported sexual aversion toward their peers" (p. 1822). Fifty-three percent reported strong or moderate sexual attraction toward at least some of their peers, and 43% reported feelings of indifference. Many interviewees, including those who felt strong sexual attraction, "saw the relationship as something 'different,' and often they could not envision full intercourse and a romantic relationship as a full option" (p. 1824).

Shor and Simchai account for these findings by citing the atmosphere of prohibition in relation to sex among peers at the kibbutz. Another important finding they reported is the prediction of degree of sexual attraction by group cohesion: the higher the group cohesion, the lower the sexual attraction.

Although the Shor and Simchai study is limited by the retrospective nature of their data, they present some cogent criticisms of the Westermarck hypothesis. The virtual absence of reports of sexual aversion suggests that one may need to modify the hypothesis to state that prolonged propinquity reduces sexual attraction rather than generates sexual aversion. The fact is that almost half the interviewees reported sexual indifference toward their kibbutzim peers—a rather large percentage for young people who are interacting with each other. And even those who reported sexual attraction for a peer felt something "different" and often could not envision sexual intercourse and a romantic relationship with that peer. As Shor and Simchai note, however, reports of aversion and disgust were reserved for thoughts about sex with siblings.

That factors other than prolonged propinquity, such as group cohesion, were shown to influence degree of sexual attraction does not contradict the (modified version) of the Westermarck hypothesis. Rather, it demonstrates the role of additional factors.

However it comes about, it is likely that the incest taboo has been selected out for the selective advantage it confers. Humans (and animals) practicing incest would be at a selective disadvantage due to decreased fitness, resulting from such factors as reduction in genetic variability and in hybrid vigor, greater probability of mutations, and the greater "power" of recessive genes.[6]

All this has to do with the *distal* function of the incest taboo. It does not tell us anything about how the distal function gets implemented at the *proximal* level of personal motives, desires, attitudes, and the like. Nor does it necessarily imply the existence of powerful incestuous impulses. It only outlines the selective advantage of an incest taboo. Given the selective advantage of not practicing incest and the selective disadvantage of engaging in incest, it is important that some proximal mechanisms be in place that minimizes the occurrence of incest. There are ample *opportunities* to carry out incest. This is especially so because of the fact that close members of the family live together for many years.

As noted, one "mechanism" suggested by Westermarck (1891) and supported by much evidence is the reduction of sexual interest and excitement accompanying prolonged propinquity and familiarity—a kind of negative imprinting. One can add the contrasting increase in sexual interest and excitement accompanying novelty, diversity, and unfamiliarity. The two together are highly adaptive insofar as they entail a decrease in sexual interest in family members and hence, decreased probability of incest, and an enhanced interest in Freud's (1912/1957) words, of "extraneous objects" outside the family.

It seems highly unlikely that nature would first select out universal powerful incestuous wishes and then add a universal taboo to prevent the enactment of these wishes and impulses. The "mechanism," suggested by Westermarck, which results in *decreasing* sexual interest with prolonged propinquity—particularly as the child becomes older and he or she becomes increasingly capable of, respectively, impregnating or becoming

---

[6]Here too the story is more complicated in that there are selective advantages and disadvantages for both inbreeding and outbreeding. I reserve discussion of this issue for later in the chapter.

pregnant—would be highly adaptive. This mechanism, along with the tendency for sexual interest to become intensified with novelty and diversity, would greatly facilitate the choice of an "extraneous object."

Critique of Mitchell's View

Mitchell posits a conflict or an antagonism between love (attachment) and desire (erotic and romantic passion), the source of which lies in our illusory need for "secure attachment." He implies that were we to give up this fantasy, we would not be motivated to degrade romance by trying to lock it in with predictability and commitment. However, the need for secure attachment is neither illusion nor fantasy, but certainly as legitimate a need as the need for erotic and romantic passion. It does not seem to me that, as Mitchell (2002) maintains, we are *motivated* to destroy the latter, that "we expend considerable effort degrading [romance]" (p. 28). Rather, the "degradation," or at least the diminution of romantic passion, is at least partly the "natural" outcome of the inherent relationship between the attachment and sexual systems, together with the fact the one's current partner is generally both one's attachment figure and one's sexual mate. This is a main thesis I propose and elaborate in the next section.

Mitchell (2002) writes that romantic passion requires "lack, desire for what one does not have" (p. 56). Pursuing the logical implication of that statement, it follows that when lack is removed and now one has what one desired and lacked, romantic passion will be reduced. One does not need any special motivation to reduce it. It seems, rather, that as Freud (1912/1957) maintains, it is in the very nature of sexuality that "an obstacle is required to heighten libido" (p. 187). Characteristic of long-term committed attachment relationships is the removal of the obstacle to which Freud refers. Seeking such a relationship does not mean that we are motivated to destroy romance or that we are expending considerable effort trying to degrade romance. It means, rather, that we have many complex conflicting needs and motives, and that it is just the case that the pursuit and achievement of attachment security often result in the dampening of sexual passion.

I propose that one does not need to invoke either the persistence of universal incestuous wishes or a motivation to "degrade romance" to account for the commonly observed split between love and desire or attachment and sexuality. Rather, partial antagonism between the two systems is the "natural" or default relationship between the two systems. Compare the factors that influence the development of attachment and those that influence sexual excitement and interest. The development of an attachment bond requires time and propinquity. In order for someone to serve as an attachment figure, he or she must be familiar and predictable. Characteristics such as novelty, unfamiliarity, and unpredictability are incompatible with the development of attachment. One does not become attached to a novel or unfamiliar figure. It is virtually an oxymoron to say that one's attachment figure is novel or unfamiliar. On the other hand, the intensity of sexual excitement seems to be reduced by familiarity and predictability and increased by novelty, unfamiliarity, and diversity—in Byron's words, by "fresh features"—and even by forbiddenness and illicitness (Kernberg, 1995). And yet, despite the incompatible factors that influence the development and expression of attachment and sexuality, in our culture at least, one's adult attachment figure is most frequently also one's sexual partner.

One needs one's spouse or romantic partner as one's attachment figure, to be familiar, predictable, and available. And yet, as noted, there is a good deal of evidence that predictability, familiarity, and availability frequently dampen the intensity of sexual interest and excitement. Thus, I am suggesting that, quite independent of any positing of universal incestuous wishes, the divergent pulls of the attachment and sexual systems go a good way toward accounting for the split between love and desire—which, I propose, is essentially a split between attachment and sexuality—that Freud wrote about and that is also commonly observed today.

One is reminded here of a phenomenon found in the animal kingdom that is referred to as the "Coolidge effect," based on the following story:

> "One day the President and Mrs. Coolidge were visiting a government farm. Soon after their arrival they were taken off on separate tours. When Mrs. Coolidge passed the chicken pens she paused to ask the man in charge if the rooster copulates more than once each day. 'Dozens of times,' was the reply. 'Please tell the President,' Mrs. Coolidge requested. When the President passed the pens and was told about the rooster, he asked, 'Same hen every time?' 'Oh no, Mr. President, a different one each time.' The President nodded slowly, then said, 'Tell that to Mrs. Coolidge.' (Bermant, 1976, pp. 76–77)

In many mammalian species, after copulating with a female and ejaculating several times, the male's sexual activity wanes and then eventually ceases. However, if a new estrous female is introduced, the male immediately begins to copulate again. Symons (1979) observes that in cattle and sheep the Coolidge effect is so strong that "the sexual limits of the experimental males have not been discovered" (p. 209). He also writes that "while males of many species are indiscriminate in that they will copulate with any estrous females of their species, they are extremely discriminating in that they recognize females individually, and they are partial to variety and prejudiced against familiarity" (p. 210).

In citing studies with animals, I run the risk of being accused of equating animal with human behavior, reducing the human to the animal, and overlooking the influences of culture and learning. The fact is, however, that one need not be reductionistic or be guilty of a facile equation of animal and human behavior in order to recognize that we are part of the animal kingdom and that many of our tendencies and behaviors are, partly at least, influenced by evolutionary natural selection. We do not seem to have much difficulty recognizing that aspects of the attachment system (e.g., proximity-seeking; the relation between a secure base and exploratory behavior) cut across a wide range of species. It would be surprising if that were not also true of the sexual system.

Furthermore, the phenomena I have been discussing, in particular, the relation between novelty and variety versus familiarity and sexual interest, have been widely and independently observed in humans (see Kinsey, Pomeroy, & Martin, 1948). The most obvious expression of this relationship is the widespread prevalence of extramarital sex. As has been observed by many, both marriage and extramarital sex have been reported in all human societies.

The relationship between variety and sexual interest is not in dispute. What is at issue is how one accounts for this and related phenomena. Are they attributable, as Freud (1912/1957) argues, to the persistence and fixation of incestuous wishes and fantasies? Are they attributable, as Mitchell (2002) proposes, to our positive motivation to "degrade" romantic sexual passion? Or, as I am arguing, are they, at least to a significant degree and in certain respects, attributable to the inherent relationship between the dynamics of the sexual and attachment systems and the integrative challenge that this relationship poses?

That sexual interest and attraction are heightened by newness and unfamiliarity and dampened by familiarity is, as noted earlier, in certain respects, highly adaptive in the original family situation insofar as it encourages the mating choice of "extraneous objects" (Freud, 1912/1957, p. 181) and discourages the "choice" of a family member. However, to the extent that these characteristics of sexuality, that is, intensification by newness and dampening by familiarity, continue to operate, they constitute potential threats to the stability and longevity of established long-term relationships. For, in such relationships, the originally "extraneous object" becomes a familiar one and others outside the relationship are now "extraneous objects toward whom sexual interest is directed." This presents challenges to a long-term relationship that need to be met if it is to be satisfactorily maintained.

One important way of meeting such challenges is the supplementation and partial replacement of sexual excitement and interest with an emotional (attachment) bond. In order for the couple to stay together as well as want to stay together, the factors of emotional support and mutual caring must be strong enough to maintain the relationship. That is, the relationship shifts somewhat away from being primarily a sexual one to being also an attachment relationship. This is not to say that sexual attraction and sexual satisfaction no longer play a part in the relationship. Although they may play less of a part, they continue to sustain the relationship. It is very likely that a combination of continuing sexual attraction (even if not as intense as during an earlier phase) and satisfaction and the establishment of mutual attachment represent the best recipe for an enduring and satisfactory relationship. However, as is commonly reported, sex is generally more important at the beginning of a relationship, and later in the relationship, emotional support and other similar factors become increasingly important.

There is also evidence that it takes about 2 years for all the major components of attachment (i.e., proximity-seeking; separation protest; safe haven; secure base; etc.) to be operative in the relationship. One way of interpreting this phenomenon is that sexual attraction often brings and holds the two adults together—what Hazan and Zeifman (1994) refer to as the "psychological tether"—for a long enough time to provide an opportunity for a strong emotional bond to form. However, the longevity of the relationship will, in large part, be determined by the couple's ability to maintain that emotional bond in the face of the relatively decreased role of sexual attraction. A good deal of evidence suggests that sensitive and responsive care, not sexual attraction, is the most accurate predictor of relationship longevity (e.g., Kotler, 1985).

The above account of the split between attachment and sexuality does not require invoking either incestuous wishes or the incest taboo. The operation of habituation goes some way to accounting for that split. However, there may be other factors that do involve the incest taboo. One such factor may be the triggering of the incest taboo as a consequence of the unconscious equation between current partner and early attachment figure. That is, insofar as one's romantic partner becomes one's attachment figure, *she takes on a role that is, in important respects, similar to the role played by mother.* This may trigger or intensify the incest taboo, which then makes it more difficult to experience partner as a sexual object—she becomes too identified with mother. The affectionate-attachment current may then be split off from the sensual-sexual current, which is safer and easier to experience with an "extraneous object" outside the home who is not one's attachment figure. It is important to note that while the incest *taboo* plays a central role in the above account, one need not invoke incest *wishes*.

INDIVIDUAL DIFFERENCES IN INTEGRATING ATTACHMENT AND SEXUALITY

Although it appears to be generally the case that as an attachment bond develops there is a relative waning of sexual excitement, it is also true that there are individual differences in the degree to which this occurs. Despite the general features of the attachment and sexual systems, some people show relative success in integrating love and desire and other relative failure. Why is this so? I noted above that in the formation of an attachment bond, current partner is "assigned" a role similar to the one that mother played. This is a general phenomenon that, in itself, does not account for individual differences in the ability to integrate attachment and sexuality. I would suggest that an important factor that does help account for individual differences in the integration of attachment and sexuality is the degree to which the individual (unconsciously) equates current partner and early parental figure and, as a consequence, activates and/or intensifies the incest taboo.

I propose further that a relative inability to shift from parent to current partner as one's primary attachment figure—an inability, I will try to show, that is characteristic of insecure patterns of attachment—increases the likelihood of unconsciously equating parental figure with current partner and therefore, interferes with the individual's ability to integrate love (attachment) and desire (sexuality). Another way to state my thesis is that the more unresolved one's attachment relationship to mother, the more one will react to current partner as a stand-in for mother and, therefore, be less able to experience one's current partner as a sexual figure. And conversely, the more one has been able to resolve the early attachment relationship and shift from mother to current partner as one's attachment figure, the less "contaminated" by earlier reaction and patterns will be one's current attachment relationship. I present some evidence below in support of my hypothesis.

Shift from Parent to Current Partner as Attachment Figure

There is little doubt that in the course of normal development, we progressively shift from parents to peers as attachment figures, generally culminating in one's romantic partner as one's primary attachment figure. My general hypothesis is that difficulty in making the transition from parent(s) to current partner as one's primary attachment figure is a central factor in generating what have been traditionally referred to as Oedipal issues, at the center of which is a relative inability to integrate the attachment and sexual aspects of romantic relationships. The relative inability to make this transition is linked to an unconscious equation between parental figure and current partner. One consequence is that not only are early attachment patterns transferred to current partners, but, because of the unconscious equation of current partner with parental figure, the current partner becomes a taboo sexual object, making it more difficult to experience sexual interest and feelings toward her.

Although, according to attachment theory, it is generally the case that, to some degree, early attachment patterns are transferred to the current partner, I suggest that the transfer occurs in a more unresolved way in individuals with insecure patterns of attachment. Because securely attached individuals are more likely to have resolved attachment issues with parents and to have successfully negotiated the developmental shift from parent to current partner as primary attachment figure, they are less likely unconsciously to equate the current partner with the parental figure and, therefore, are less likely to respond sexually to the current partner as a forbidden incestuous object. Contrastingly, almost by definition, avoidant and enmeshed or preoccupied individuals react to the current partner as if he or she were the parental figure. For example, if one continues to be avoidant toward the current partner, one is continuing to react defensively, as if one were experiencing the current partner as rejecting or intrusive, similar to the way one experienced the early parental figure.

Latchaw (2010) investigated the relationship between attachment pattern and evidence of unresolved Oedipal conflicts. Based on the literature, Oedipal conflicts were operationally defined in terms of achievement anxiety, fear of intimacy, sexual attitudes, hypercompetitive attitudes, difficulty integrating sex with love, and a history of triangular relationships. A composite score of these "Oedipal" measures was significantly positively related to insecure attachment and significantly negatively related to secure attachment. The most robust relationships were found between dismissing and fearful attachment and fear of intimacy, and both dismissive and anxious attachment and sexual conflict.

Consider first the avoidant pattern. That one continues to be avoidant toward current partner strongly suggests that one is continuing to react defensively, as if one were experiencing at some level current partner as rejecting and/or intrusive, similar to the way one experienced the early parental figure. One would expect that due to this unconscious equation of current partner with early parental figure, the avoidantly attached individual will have greater difficulty integrating sexuality and attachment. Indeed, there is a good deal of evidence suggesting that avoidantly attached individuals tend to separate sexual from attachment feelings. For example, Feeney and Noller (1990) have reported that university students classified as avoidant are more likely to endorse acceptance of multiple relationships, limited involvement and commitment, and the use of sex for fun rather than as an expression of emotional depth. They are also more likely to express jealousy of sexual infidelity rather than emotional infidelity (Levy & Kelly, 2010).

As noted, Latchaw (2010) found a significant relationship between avoidant attachment and fear of intimacy as well as presence of sexual conflict. In short, avoidant individuals seem to be characterized by relative difficulty in establishing and maintaining an attachment bond as well as a relative disjunction between sex and attachment—both of which are not especially conducive to the longevity of romantic relationships.

Although they show a different pattern than the avoidantly attached, anxiously attached individuals also tend to react more to the current partner as if she were the parental figure. That is, they expect inconsistency in the availability of the current attachment figure and are preoccupied with fears of abandonment—just as they were in relation to the early parental figure. Thus, in common with the avoidantly attached, to the extent that they also unconsciously equate current partner with parental figure, they are also more likely to have greater difficulty integrating sexuality and attachment. Evidence supporting this inference includes findings that, more than the securely or avoidantly attached, anxiously attached individuals report seeking support from someone other than their partner; report frequent and intense love experiences; report rapid physical and emotional involvement; fall in love more often; and report more "love at first sight" experiences (Feeney & Noller, 1990). They are also high in sexual conflict (Latchaw, 2010).

If one can say that the avoidantly attached emphasize sexuality "at the expense of" attachment, one can correspondingly say that the enmeshed/preoccupied emphasize attachment "at the expense of" sexuality. That is, their sexual behavior and experience seem to be largely in the service of repeatedly attempting to gain reassurance that they will not be abandoned. An interesting finding that supports this view is that compared to securely attached individuals, who report a fairly stable level of satisfaction with their romantic relationship, the reported level of satisfaction of anxiously attached individuals tends to vary with whether they have had a recent sexual interaction with their partner (Davis, Shaver, & Vernon, 2004). For the latter, the sexual interaction seems to serve a reassuring function. For example, Davis et al. (2004) found that an attachment style characterized by attachment anxiety "was positively related to reports of interest in sex being higher when feeling insecure about the relationship" (p. 1083). They also found that attachment anxiety was significantly associated with different motives for sex (e.g., manipulation, stress reduction), but that "the largest of these associations were between attachment anxiety and the motives of reassurance ... and emotional closeness" (p. 1084). There is also evidence that women's agreement to unwanted sex is often motivated by the fear of rejection and abandonment associated with anxious attachment (Davis, Follette, & Vernon, 2001).[7]

A number of other findings link attachment patterns and sexual behavior. For example, Bogaert and Sadava (2002) found that compared to anxiously attached women, securely attached women were more likely to have fewer sexual partners and to be older at age of first sexual intercourse.

Similar to Davis et al. (2004), Impett and Peplau (2002) reported that anxiously attached women were most likely to consent to unwanted sex in a hypothetical scenario out of concern that their partner might lose interest in them for failure to comply with the request for sex. Avoidantly attached women were also more likely than securely attached women to consent to unwanted sex in order to fulfill relationship obligations and to avoid conflict.

ATTACHMENT PATTERNS AND INFIDELITY

A number of studies have also been done on infidelity and attachment patterns. Although Weisberger (2000) reported no differences among attachment styles in the likelihood of individuals with different attachment styles to behave unfaithfully or to be involved with someone who had behaved unfaithfully, a number of studies have reported that insecure attachment is, indeed, correlated with infidelity (Blumstein & Schwartz, 1983; Bogaert & Sadava, 2002; Thompson, 1983). Allen and Baucom (2004) found that

---

[7]Although I have been discussing different attachment patterns as if they were pure types, it is likely that many people have access to multiple attachment patterns that are likely to be hierarchically arranged and differentially elicited in different interactional situations. The idea of a hierarchical arrangement suggests a dominant pattern that is more or less characteristic of the individual. I think this is likely to be the case for most people. Furthermore, maladaptive and troubled relationships, particularly maladaptive intimate relationships, seem to be characterized by rigidity and repetitiveness of (insecure) attachment pattern—which is but one aspect of the general rigidity, repetitiveness, and "adhesiveness" of pathological behavior.

whereas avoidant–dismissives reported engaging in extradyadic intimacy (EDI) in response to a need for space and freedom in their primary relationship, enmeshed–preoccupied and avoidant–fearfuls reported engaging in EDI out of feelings of neglect and a desire to be cared for. Avoidant-dismissive men reported more infidelity than any other group, and overall, men cheated more than women. Finally, enmeshed–preoccupied women reported more infidelity over the prior 2 years than securely attached women.

In a study by Cohen (2005), fidelity was measured using a newly constructed Scale of Relational Infidelity (SORI). (This name was changed to read "SORI" on the copy distributed to participants, so as not to appear too threatening.) This 26-item scale requires participants to respond to a number of questions concerning physical and emotional acts in which they have engaged with someone other than their significant other while in a monogamous relationship. There are four sections to this scale—constituting 13 questions—addressing physical forms of infidelity, romantic extradyadic forays (cybersex, dating, flirting, etc.), extradyadic sexual fantasies, and extradyadic emotional fantasies. The questions in each section comprise four spectrums, each of which begins with the most benign form of infidelity and gradually increases to more overt forms of infidelity.

Cohen (2005) found that for both men and women, compared to avoidantly attached individuals, securely attached individuals reported lower levels of infidelity. Other findings included a significant positive association between secure attachment and relationship satisfaction and a significant negative association between relationship satisfaction and reported infidelity. Another interesting finding was that individuals who perceived partners as preoccupied or fearful avoidant reported the highest level of infidelity.

In addition to the studies that I have described, there is also much clinical material that sheds light on the relation between the attachment and sexual systems. It is not at all uncommon in clinical work to deal with patients who report a split between love and desire as a central feature of their intimate relationships. I worked with a patient who had an intense sexual aversion toward his wife and, at the same time, clearly experienced her as an attachment figure who served as a kind of psychic organizer for him (in Kohut's term, an archaic self object). Because his wife had become unconsciously equated with his mother, this man seemed incapable of sexual feelings toward her. He reported shuddering in disgust both when his elderly mother embraced and kissed him and when he thought of having sex with his wife.

Another patient reported that although he was not especially sexually attracted to her, he chose his wife because she was everything his mother was not, reliable, supportive, and accepting—that is, unlike his mother, a good attachment figure (although, of course, he did not use that term). However, problems soon arose when he found women outside the marriage sexually exciting and his wife sexually uninteresting—although she unquestioningly remained his attachment figure. Because she remained his attachment figure, he could not fully separate from her. Instead he attempted to both maintain his relationship with his wife and carry on a separate sexual life, a not uncommon situation, but one that caused him and his wife great distress.

In my view, Freud would be correct if he maintained that in the above cases the wife recalls the forbidden incestuous figure, but would not be correct in assuming an incestuous fixation on mother. That is, I believe that because my patient unconsciously equates wife with mother the incest taboo is triggered, with the result that he cannot feel sexual toward her. This is different from saying that because his wife elicits forbidden incestuous wishes, he cannot feel sexual toward her. I am suggesting the operation of an incest taboo without positing persistent incestuous wishes. I believe that my patient's need to find an adequate attachment figure who would replace the inadequate one his mother represented worked to preclude strong sexual interest and excitement.

As we have seen, in his discussion of "psychical impotence," Freud (1912/1957) writes about the individual's inability to combine the "affectionate and sensual currents." Interpreted literally, this means that where individuals feel affection, they cannot feel sensual and sexual, and where they feel sensual and sexual, they cannot feel affection. But my patient could feel *neither* affectionate *nor* sexual feelings toward his wife, but did experience *both* affectionate and sexual feelings with his mistress.[8] In this particular case, the split between love and desire was not characterized by a general inability to combine the "affectionate and sensual currents," but by an inability to experience either affectionate or sexual feelings toward *the specific woman equated with mother* (i.e., his wife). Perhaps affection is too close to sexuality for it to be safely experienced toward the taboo object.

Hence, in the case of this patient, it is more accurate to refer to a split between the attachment and sexual systems rather than the affectionate

---

[8]Of course, my patient was able to feel both affectionate and sexual toward his mistress as long as she remained his mistress and did not assume the role of wife. There is evidence throughout his relationship with his mistress that his sexual interest in her has waned when he has seriously considered leaving his wife and making a commitment to his mistress—not an uncommon pattern.

and sensual currents. For, although my patient did not experience either affection or sexual feelings toward his wife, there is no question that he experienced her as his attachment figure.

Furthermore, I do not think this is an unusual pattern. My impression is that one sees such a pattern not infrequently in clinical work. It is likely that, when extreme, insecure attachment patterns may preclude free feelings of affection as well as sexuality toward the attachment figure. There is too much anxiety, conflict and ambivalence, and defensiveness in relation to both the early and current attachment figure.

Thus, although up to this point, I have used these terms interchangeably, I think the real failure in "psychical impotence," and in the split between love and desire may lie not so much in the person's inability to combine what Freud (1912/1957) referred to as the "affectionate and sensual currents," but rather in his or her inability to combine feelings linked to attachment and sexuality.

ATTACHMENT AND ADULT SEXUALITY

Gender Differences

Let me turn to the issue of gender differences, which has been hovering over the entire discussion of attachment and sexuality. As noted earlier, Freud (1912/1957) does include women as well as men in his account of the split between love and desire. Thus, in commenting on the failure to experience pleasure, he refers to "the immense number of frigid women" (p. 185) paralleling "psychoanesthetic" men (p. 184). He also refers to women who are frigid in their relationship with their spouse, but show a "capacity ... for normal sensation as soon as the condition for prohibition is re-established by a secret love-affair: unfaithful to their husband, they are able to keep a second order of faith with their lover" (p. 186). However, by far, most of Freud's discussion concerns men.[9]

The gender issue comes especially to the fore in Freud's formulation of the role of infantile sexuality in object choice. The fact is that for both men and women, the caregiver is almost always a woman, mother. If however,

---

[9]Another issue that hovers over the entire discussion and that has not been covered is the question of homosexuality. Does the relationship between attachment and sexuality that I have formulated apply to homosexuality as well as heterosexuality? There are also questions of gender within a homosexual orientation that need to be considered. For example, does the relationship between novelty and sexual arousal hold equally for male and female homosexuality? My impression is that it does not. However, there is simply little research on the relationship between attachment and sexuality in homosexual relationships. This is clearly a research gap that needs to be filled.

the earliest infantile sexuality and love experiences determine the prototype of one's object choice, it is mother who should represent that prototype for both men and women. But this conclusion conflicts with the Oedi-
pally based prediction that it is the prototype of opposite sex parent that
constitutes the basis for object choice. On that view, for women, father, not
mother, would represent the prototype.

Why is father rather than mother the object choice for the little girl?
To answer this question, Freud (1925b/1961) weaves a complex speculative
narrative that contains the following elements: The little girl observes that
she does not have a penis. Her resentment against her mother "who sent
her into the world so insufficiently equipped" leads to "a loosening of the
girl's relation with her mother as a love object" (p. 254). The next step is
that the girl "gives up her wish for a penis and puts in place of it a wish for
a child: and *with that purpose in view* she takes her father as a love-object"
(p. 256).

The above narrative is utterly speculative and is supported by little or
no empirical evidence. As Strachey (Freud, 1925b/1961) makes clear, "From
early days Freud made complaints of the obscurity enveloping the sexual
life of women" (p. 243). He also notes, "over a long period from the time of
the Dora analysis in 1900, Freud's interest had not been directed to femi-
nine psychology" (p. 245), and he also observes that Freud "assume[d] very
often that the psychology of women could be taken simply as analogous to
that of men" (p. 244). However, Freud had to withdraw that assumption
and substituted for it the convoluted narrative that I have briefly outlined
above. At various points, Freud acknowledged that "we know less about
the sexual life of little girls than of boys" (Freud, 1926b/1959, p. 212)
and stated that he was puzzled by and did not understand female sexuality, which he variously refers to as "an impenetrable obscurity" (Freud,
1933/1964, p. 151)—as "a dark continent" (Freud, 1926b/1959, p. 212)
and an "enigma of wonder" (Freud, 1933/1964, p. 137)—interesting choice
of words. In short, one should perhaps not expect Freud's formulations to
shed much light on the nature of female sexuality.

There are likely to be gender differences not only with regard to the
nature of sexuality, but also with regard to the nature of the relationship
between attachment and sexuality. As discussed earlier, Diamond (2003)
(see also Fisher, 1998) has proposed that "desire is governed by the *sexual
mating* system" (p. 174), the goal of which is reproduction, whereas romantic love (Diamond is clearly referring to long-term intimate relationships) is
governed by the *attachment* or *pair-bonding* system ... the goal of which
is the maintenance of an enduring association" (p. 174) for the purpose of

survival of dependent offspring. Diamond also suggests that pair-bonding or attachment originally evolved, not in the context of sexual mating but instead "exploited" the already existing infant–caregiver attachment system "for the new purpose of maintaining associations between adult reproductive partners" (p. 174).

Although both men and women have a profound interest in maintaining the pair-bond for the purpose of protection and survival of dependent offspring, from the pure perspective of propagating one's genes, it is the woman who has made the greater investment during nine months of pregnancy and it is the woman who is certain of the progeny of her offspring. Furthermore, the man can propagate his genes through impregnating an indefinite number of women. Hence, as far as inclusive fitness is concerned (Trivers, 1971), compared to men, women are more likely to emphasize attachment over sexual motives. They are likely to have a greater investment in providing stability and protection for their limited offspring.

There are other differences worth noting. The effects of novelty and unfamiliarity on sexual interest and excitement seem to be more pronounced in males than females. For example, the so-called Coolidge effect appears to be limited to males—although, as far as I know, no one has investigated female sexual arousal as a function of novelty and unfamiliarity in animals. From a clinical perspective, it is quite common in work with couples to find the husband complaining that following the entry of children into the family, the wife is neither as emotionally nor sexually available as she was prior to the birth of children. It is as if he is complaining that there has been a shift from the wife's primary investment in the couple to a primary investment in the child or children. It is interesting to observe, in this regard, that the greatest possibility of divorce is at three years of marriage, a point at which there is a greater likelihood of offspring survival.

Following divorce or separation, not only is it far more common for children to remain with mother than father, but also far more common for mother to *want* to retain physical custody, even though this circumstance may decrease her chances for a new relationship. My specific point here is to note the differential investment in offspring between men and women and its potential impact on the relationship between attachment and sexuality.

Attachment and Sexuality in Mate Choice

Freud argued that one important expression of the Oedipus complex is the choice of a mate based on a prototype of one's parental figure. He asserts that "there can be no doubt that every object-choice whatever is based ... on these prototypes. A man, especially, looks for someone who can represent his picture of his mother" (Freud, 1905/1953, p. 228). He also writes that the object will "still be chosen on the model (imago) of the infantile ones" (Freud, 1912/1957, p. 181). One should note that the choice of a mate based on a prototype of one's parental figure does not in itself necessarily support an Oedipal interpretation. The choice could be due to factors other than the presumed persistence of incestuous wishes.

Two questions need to be raised regarding Freud's formulation. One, do people and animals, in fact, tend to select mates who are similar to parental figures? And two, if this is the case, what are the factors involved in such choices? With regard to the first question there is evidence that both animals and humans tend to choose a mate who is similar but not identical to those with whom they were reared. For example, in one study quail preferred members of the opposite sex who were first cousins to those who were third cousins, siblings, and unrelated (Bateson, 1982). And mice, too, show greatest sexual interest in mates of intermediate relatedness, often second cousins (Barnard & Aldhous, 1991; Barnard & Fitzimmons, 1988). There is also evidence from bird and rodent species that these animals avoid mating with close kin but tend to choose mates who are similar in appearance.

A similar pattern, referred to as positive assortative mating, is found in humans (e.g., Bereczkei et al., 2002; Zajonc et al., 1987). That is, people tend to select mates who are similar to themselves (and therefore, presumably similar to family members) in physical, social, and psychological characteristics. In a *New York Times* article on Iraqi marriages, the reporter, John Tierney (2003) notes that nearly half the marriages in Iraq are to first or second cousins. He writes that "cousin marriages were once the norm throughout the world" (p. 12) and reports an interview with an Iraqi woman who responded to her uncle's proposal that she marry his son by stating, "I was a little surprised, but I knew right away it was a wise choice. It is *safer* (my italics) to marry a cousin than a stranger" (p. 1). Tierney cites the anthropologist Robin Fox's point that in much of the world people are divided into two groups: kin and strangers; and as the Iraqi woman's comment suggests, kin are safer.

Thus, there appears to be evidence that both animals and humans tend to select mates who, if not similar specifically to parental figures, are at least similar to family members. We can now turn to the second question, namely, what might be the basis for this phenomenon? If the Westermarck hypothesis that familiarity dampens sexual attraction holds, one would expect diminished sexual attraction, not only to family members, but also, through a process of generalization, to possible mates who are similar to family members. That is, if a mechanism for incest avoidance is the inhibition or diminution of sexual desire that is associated with familial attachment, then why would one tend to select a mate who is similar to family members? Why not select as dissimilar a mate as possible? A number of answers to these questions have been offered. Bateson (1983) has proposed a theory of "optimal outbreeding," which predicts that animals are likely to "select a mate with an intermediate degree of [genetic] relatedness so that the costs of inbreeding and outbreeding are balanced and minimized" (Morehead, 1999, p. 360).

Bateson's theory of optimal outbreeding constitutes a "distal" explanation of the phenomenon in question. That is, it focuses on the ultimate evolutionary functions of the behavior. It does not, however, tell us what the "proximal" mechanisms and factors are likely to be. Thus, when an animal selects a mate of an intermediate degree of relatedness, it is not likely to be proximally motivated by the desire to balance the costs of outbreeding and inbreeding. And when we prefer as a mate someone who is similar to ourselves along physical, psychological, and social dimensions, we are certainly not responding on the basis of distal selection advantages, but rather in terms of proximal personal factors.

What might these proximal personal factors be? I would suggest that paralleling the distal factor of balancing inbreeding and outbreeding costs is the proximal factor of balancing sexual attraction and feelings of comfort, safety, and familiarity, with familiarity being especially important in increasing the likelihood for the eventual formation of an attachment bond. One must keep in mind that, as Fox (1980) has pointed out, there is a distinction between sexual attraction and mate selection. Although sexual attraction is often an important factor in mate selection, other factors are likely to be involved. The choice of a mate on the basis of optimal similarity makes sense insofar as it permits *both* sexual feelings *and* attachment feelings. Optimal similarity would be just what one would expect if choice of mate were made on the basis of an unconscious "best fit compromise" between sexual interest and potential for an enduring attachment bond.

The choice of a mate who is very dissimilar to family members might maximize sexual interest, but render the formation of an attachment bond more difficult. Conversely, the choice of a mate who is too similar to family members might maximize the formation of an attachment bond but, in accord with the Westermarck hypothesis, make sexual interest and excitement more difficult. So, a choice made on the basis of optimal similarity seems to represent the optimal compromise between the somewhat conflicting "demands" of the sexual and attachment systems.

In short, I propose the hypothesis that mate selection on the basis of optimal similarity to kin represents a "best fit" compromise between the pulls and demands of the sexual and attachment systems. It is responsive to (1) incest avoidance and (2) feelings of relative comfort because the mate is experienced as familiar, safe, and redolent of family members, including one's attachment figure. Hence, it permits *both* sexual feelings *and* attachment feelings.

There is still another reason that optimal similarity may constitute the best basis for mate selection. In an entirely different context from the current discussion, Gaines (1997) has discussed two different kinds of object choice: one in which the new object is very similar to parental figures and characterized by rigid repetition of early maladaptive patterns with parent, and the other in which the new object is sufficiently similar to parental figures so that old patterns and responses will be triggered, but also sufficiently different to permit mastery, reworking of old patterns, and the development of new patterns and a more gratifying relationship. So, from a somewhat different perspective, optimal similarity also emerges as the most adaptive basis for the choice of mate.

I would suggest the additional hypothesis that choices made on the basis of optimal similarity are more likely to be associated with greater relationship longevity and satisfaction. Although the relation between optimal similarity and relationship longevity has not been systematically investigated, Thiessen and Gregg (1980) cite evidence that similar mates show increased levels of fertility and longer, more stable relationships.

I would also predict that securely attached individuals are more likely to make optimally similar mate choices than those who are insecurely attached. The latter, I would hypothesize, are more likely to choose mates who are either very similar or very different from family members. One can speculate that anxiously attached individuals will be more likely to choose mates who are very similar to family members and avoidant–dismissive individuals are more likely to choose mates who are very different from family members. Or, perhaps, the issue is not only the actual degree of similarity between mate and family members, but also how similar or different the mate is *experienced* by the individual. One might expect that, in accord with their respective attachment patterns and strategies, the anxiously attached individual will consciously and unconsciously experience his or her partner as very similar to early family members (particularly, the early attachment figure), and that the avoidant–dismissive individual will consciously experience his or her partner as very different from his or her attachment figure and unconsciously experience his or her partner as similar to his or her early attachment figure. These predictions can be empirically investigated.[10]

SUMMARY AND RECAPITULATION

To sum up my central arguments, I have suggested that not only is there a degree of functional independence between the attachment and sexual systems, but also a natural or default partial antagonism between the two systems. That is, whereas sexual interest and excitement are enhanced by novelty, unfamiliarity, and related features, attachment requires familiarity and predictability. And yet, as adults, one's attachment figure is also most frequently one's sexual partner. Given the operation of these two systems, as one's current partner becomes one's attachment figure, sexual interest and excitement are likely to wane, a prediction that is generally supported by empirical evidence. This state of affairs presents the individual with an integrative challenge that is met by different individuals with varying degrees of success.

I have suggested that an important factor in determining the individual's degree of success in integrating love and desire or attachment and sexuality lies in his or her ability to differentiate between parent and current partner as his attachment figure. A relative failure to accomplish this integration is associated with an unconscious equation between parent and current partner, with the result that the current partner also becomes a taboo sexual object, just as the parent was. If, as the Westermarck hypothesis and the evidence I have cited suggests, there is a kind of sexual negative imprinting toward members of one's family, then the greater the degree to which the current partner becomes equated with the former, the greater

---

[10]The distinction made earlier between actual similarity and experienced similarity between mate and family members suggests the operation of the process of transference familiar to psychodynamic theorists and clinicians, which needs to be taken into account if one is to more fully understand the relation between the individual's experience of current relationships and relationships with early parental figures. I am referring to a familiar process in couples, particularly troubled couples, by which the partner is unconsciously transformed into the early parental figure. This unconscious transforming process includes both the individual's unconscious experience of his partner as if she were his parent as well as his tendency, through his own behavior, to induce and elicit behaviors and responses from his partner that are, in fact, similar to responses from early parental figures.

the difficulty in experiencing sexual feelings toward the current partner. In some cases, this can even take the form of sexual aversion.

I have also argued that compared to secure attachment, insecure patterns of attachment are characterized by a relative failure to shift from parent to current partner as attachment figure. Hence, one would expect that insecurely attached individuals would have greater difficulty integrating feelings linked to attachment and sexuality—that is, would have greater difficulty having sexual feelings toward their attachment figure. And, indeed, the evidence I have cited suggests that, albeit in different ways, this is the case for both avoidant and anxiously attached individuals.

In short, the split between love and desire, a phenomenon that for Freud was at the core of Oedipal conflicts, can be profitably understood in terms of the general relation between the attachment and sexual systems as well as the individual vicissitudes in dealing with the competing pulls and demands of these two motivational systems. I have also tried to show that the split between love and desire can be accounted for without positing universal powerful incestuous wishes, which is at the core of Freud's account of the Oedipus complex. I have also discussed gender differences with regard to the relationship between attachment and sexuality. And finally, I have suggested that choice of mate can be understood as a compromise between attachment and sexual motives.

CHAPTER 9

Attachment and Aggression

Before embarking on a discussion of attachment and aggression, a distinction needs to be made between what one might refer to as a non-hostile aggression in the service of territoriality, hunting, sexual competition, and protection of the young, and aggression in the form of anger and hostility. As someone strongly influenced by ethology, Bowlby was surely aware of this distinction and likely took it for granted. In his discussion of aggression, anger, and hostility, Bowlby consistently viewed them as relative to threats to the attachment bond. It is no accident that the title of Volume 2 in his trilogy is not "Attachment and Loss, Separation: Anxiety, and *Aggression*," but rather "Attachment and Loss, Separation: Anxiety and *Anger*." Hence, references to aggression in this chapter mainly refer to hostility and anger.

Bowlby's conceptualization and discussion of aggression reveal with particular clarity his differences with the views of Freud and Klein, especially Klein. Their conceptions of the nature of aggression are but one expression, albeit a particularly clear one, of their differences regarding the relative emphasis on the endogenous factors of inborn drive and fantasy versus actual events and experiences of threat, separation, and loss. Bowlby consistently rejects Klein's positing of an inborn death instinct or destructive drive. Instead, he consistently attributes anger and aggressive behavior to environmental events and "real-life" experiences such as loss and separation.

In his review of the psychoanalytic literature on separation anxiety (Appendix I) of Volume 2, Bowlby (1973) rejects Klein's view that the death instinct is the primary cause of anxiety and that neurotic anxiety "derives from the infant's apprehension that the loved mother has been destroyed by his sadistic impulses" (Klein, Heimann, Isaacs, & Rivière, 1952, p. 288); or that "when [an infant] misses [his mother], and his needs are not satisfied her absence is felt to be the result of his destructive impulses" (Klein et al., 1952, p. 87). He also rejects Klein's insistence that "increased anxiety is always both increased by and caused by increased hostility" (Bowlby, p. 255). Bowlby (1969/1982) also characterizes Klein's view in the following way: "all aggressive feeling and behavior is an expression of a death instinct that wells up within and must be directed outward" (p. 254).

In striking contrast to Klein's formulation, Bowlby repeatedly views anger and hostility not as primary, but as reactions to separation and loss and to the caregiver's unresponsiveness and/or inaccessibility. As Bowlby simply puts it, the child's behavior is an "expression of anger at the way he has been treated" (p. 246). These reactions may take the form of protest (i.e., to loss or abandonment) and may be preceded by longing, anxiety, and guilt. He approvingly describes Fairbairn's position as maintaining that "in the absence of frustration … , an infant would not direct aggression against his love object." What leads him to do so is—and here Bowlby quotes from Fairbairn—"deprivation and frustration in his libidinal relationships—and more particularly … the trauma of separation from his mother" (Bowlby, p. 255). In short, in contrast to a discharge model of aggression, Bowlby along with Fairbairn, adopts a frustration–aggression hypothesis.

As noted in Chapter 1, one of Bowlby's formative clinical experiences was his work with delinquent boys, which culminated in his monograph *Forty-Four Juvenile Thieves* (Bowlby, 1944). This experience appears to have been an important influence in developing his conception of aggression in the form of anger, hostility, and antisocial behavior as largely attributable to early neglect, maltreatment, loss, separation, and threat of separation. That is, aggression is elicited by threats to the attachment bond.

In the course of his writings, Bowlby (1980) provides many other examples of both children and adults reacting to separation and loss with anger and hostility. He cites a study by Heinicke (1956) and by Heinicke and Westheimer (1966) in which children in a residential nursery exhibited more "violent hostility" (p. 13) than children in a day nursery. As for adults, Bowlby cites the work of Parkes documenting the frequency of anger in recent widows. This anger could take the form of general irritability or anger at specific persons, including the dead husband. Bowlby views such anger "as an intelligible constituent of the urgent though fruitless effort a bereaved person is making to restore the bond that has been severed. So long as anger continues, it seems, loss is not being accepted as permanent and hope is still lingering on" (p. 91).

A COMPARISON OF AGGRESSION IN ATTACHMENT THEORY AND CONTEMPORARY PSYCHOANALYTIC THEORIES

Although Bowlby's disagreements were, of course, mainly with Freudian and Kleinian theory—the dominant psychoanalytic theories of his day— how do his views on aggression compare with the contemporary psychoanalytic theories of self psychology and American relational psychoanalysis? Similar to Bowlby, self psychology also views aggression primarily as reactive rather than inborn. However, according to Kohut (e.g., 1984), anger and rage are attributable mainly to the individual's experience of narcissistic injury rather than to a threat to the attachment bond. In a certain sense, one can perhaps construe narcissistic injury as a threat to the attachment bond insofar as such injury is experienced when the selfobject is not providing support in shoring up the individual's self-cohesiveness. However, that construal may perhaps be forcing an alignment between self psychology and attachment theory. For the fact is that, whereas Bowlby views anger in response to threat as motivated by the attempt to restore the attachment bond, Kohut tends to view anger and rage as an "automatic" effect of self-fragmentation brought about by selfobject failures.

Mitchell's (1993) position on the origin and nature of aggression is quite nuanced. He contrasts the two traditional theoretical positions regarding the nature of aggression: (1) aggression as a primary drive, a position associated with Freud and Klein and (2) aggression as a "secondary" reaction to such experiences as helplessness, anxiety, frustration, and ego weakness. Mitchell's own view is much closer to the second position insofar as he rejects the idea of aggression as a "propulsive" force that needs to be discharged. However, he recognizes the biological basis for a capacity for aggression and the ubiquitousness of aggression.

This latter position seems to be entirely in accord with an attachment theory perspective. However, similar to Kohut, Mitchell (1993) sees a threat to the "endangered self" as the primary precipitant of aggression. And further, because "endangerment is an unalterable and perpetual feature of human existence" (p. 171), aggression is inevitable and in each of us there is a "destructive version of the self" (p. 171) with which we have to live. Furthermore, overlooked by most theories of aggression, according to Mitchell, is "the constructive, arousing, enlivening feature of hostility" (p. 171). Hence, for Mitchell, the ideal goal of treatment is not to end with "I am a basically loving person who sometimes, atypically, gets angry and hateful when threatened" (p. 171). "Such an ending," according to Mitchell, "leaves out too much and smoothes over a great deal that is potentially vitalizing and enriching in aggressive experience" (p. 171). Rather, a "more ideal ending involves a sense that "I exist in different states of mind at different times, some loving, some hateful" (p. 171).

It seems to me that in pointing to the "constructive, enlivening, vitalizing, and enriching" nature of aggression, Mitchell may be sloughing over important differences between nondestructive aggression and destructive and hostile aggression. However, most important in the present context, although, as noted, there is a good deal of convergence between certain aspects of Mitchell's view of aggression and an attachment theory perspective, there is little in attachment theory that is hospitable to the idea that in each of us there is "a destructive version of the self" and that aggression—at least in the form of hostility—is "potentially vitalizing and enlivening." About the closest one can get in attachment theory to Mitchell's view of aggression as potentially constructive is Bowlby's (1973, 1980) idea that certain forms of the child's angry reaction to abandonment are "functional" in the sense that they may discourage such behavior on the part of the caregiver.

Among contemporary psychoanalytic theorists who view themselves as object relations theorists, Kernberg (e.g., 1976, 1980, 2005) is one of the few who accepts a version of traditional drive theory and who "believe[s] that libidinal and aggressive drive derivatives are invested in object relations from very early in life" (Kernberg, 2005, p. 67). According to Kernberg, the infant's early affective interactions with caregiver are divided or split into "good" and "bad" object and self-representations and accompanying affects. That is, the "good" experiences (e.g., "the sensuous gratifications of the satisfied baby at the breast" [Kernberg]) are internalized as positive representations of object and self associated with positive affect states. "Bad" experiences (e.g., pain, frustration, deprivation) are separately internalized with negative affect states such as fear and rage. According to Kernberg, splitting between "good" and "bad" representations and accompanying affect states is a normal process early in life.

In normal development, over time the child integrates these split representations and affects, thereby achieving object constancy, a relatively stable self and ego organization, and relative affect stability. Under certain pathogenic conditions, the child is not able to develop beyond the use of splitting or regresses to the use of splitting as a major defense. According to Kernberg (2005) such is the case in borderline personality organization. The primary function of splitting, according to Kernberg, is to keep one's negative representations and affect states from contaminating one's positive representations and affect states with the consequence that one's mental life is saturated primarily with painful negative and destructive experiences and representations.

One way to describe the above state of affairs is to say that one must keep one's destructive rage and hostility away from positive representations lest the latter be destroyed. According to Kernberg (1993), for some individuals intensely destructive rage is largely a product of constitutional endowment of excessive aggression; and for some intense aggression is due to excessive frustration and deprivation; or to an interaction between constitutional endowment and negative life experiences.

It is difficult to locate where on the theoretical spectrum Kernberg's theorizing belongs. As we can see from the above, his formulations contain elements of both a drive discharge model and a frustration–aggression hypothesis. Despite Kernberg's endorsement of drive theory, there are a number of points of contact between Kernberg's view of aggression and that of attachment theory:

1. There is a "family resemblance" between Kernberg's concepts of object and self-representations and characteristic affect and Bowlby's concept of internal working model.
2. Kernberg's idea that the child needs to keep negative representations and affects from contaminating his or her positive representations and affects is similar, in certain respects, to the idea found in both Fairbairn's object relations theory and attachment theory that parental idealization is motivated by the individual's need to (a) ward off painful affect states and (b) preserve the attachment bond. This pattern is particularly characteristic of the avoidantly attached individual who employs parental idealization as a defense and who shows evidence of contradictory multiple working models that are split off from each other. Indeed, both avoidant and disorganized classifications in infant are predictive of dissociation in adolescence and young adulthood (Dozier, Chase, Stovall-McClough, & Albus, 2008).

This finding poses somewhat of a problem insofar as, according to Kernberg, (1) splitting is most characteristic of borderline conditions and (2) it is preoccupied attachment (as well as unresolved) rather than avoidant attachment that is most frequently associated with borderline conditions (e.g., Adam, Sheldon-Keller, & West, 1996; Agrawal, Gunderson, Holmes, & Lyons-Ruth, 2004). Clearly, further research is needed in this area. For example, one would want to know whether what is referred to as dissociation is truly dissociation or *repression*, which, according to Kernberg, is quite different from dissociation or splitting.

There is perhaps one important difference between attachment theory and Kernberg's views of aggression, which suggests substantially different versions of the frustration–aggression hypothesis. According to Kernberg (1980), aggression is, so to speak, a default "automatic" response to frustration. To the extent that it is motivated, the motives for aggression are primarily to remove the obstacles that frustrate one's goals and, on occasion, to destroy the source of frustration. From Kernberg's psychoanalytic perspective, the goal emphasized is drive gratification of some kind. From an attachment theory perspective, the goal emphasized has to do with maintaining the attachment bond. Hence, in this case, removing the obstacles that frustrate one's goals would mean removing the barriers to maintaining an attachment bond. And, of course, this is precisely what Bowlby (1973, 1980) argues when he notes that anger and aggression in response to separation, loss, and abandonment are intended to convey the message "do not do this again" and thereby preserve the attachment bond. Thus, for Bowlby, destroying the object could not normally be one of the motives for aggression insofar as it would contradict the primary aim of anger, namely, preserving and maintaining the attachment bond. One can speculate that, according to attachment theory, only in states of utter despair and hopelessness would destruction of the object emerge as a primary motive for aggression.

AGGRESSION AND THE ATTACHMENT BOND

As noted, according to Bowlby (1973), the primary adaptive functions of anger and protest in response to separation and loss is that they serve as an aid in reunion to the attachment figure and in discouraging further separations. Bowlby cited a number of studies supporting his hypothesis, including, as noted, the evidence that young children (13 to 32 months of age) in a residential nursery were more aggressive than children who stayed at home (Heinicke, 1956; Heinicke & Westheimer, 1966), and that the delinquent's anger is elicited by threats of separation.[1] However, anger as a response

---

[1] Bowlby (1973) cites other examples of adaptive aggression. For example, he cites evidence that the dominant male baboon acts aggressively toward members of his group when he sights a predator. Such aggression induces fear, which then activates the attachment system, thus serving the protective function of keeping members of the group from wandering off.

to separation and loss becomes maladaptive when (1) the anger continues too long and (2) most important, when the anger attenuates and further threatens the attachment bond, for example, by triggering the attachment figure's counter anger.

One frequently observes in clinical work the operation of maladaptive hostility in response to threats to the attachment bond. For example, in the case of a woman with whom I worked, her relationship with her husband was characterized by a repetitive pattern in which her experiences of rejection, humiliation, and emotional unavailability on his part triggered uncontrollable rage and determination to leave the relationship. Her rage reliably triggered his rejection and his threat to end the relationship. In my patient this triggered anxiety, an unbearable sense of loss, despair, suicidal feelings, and an emotional conviction that she could not survive without him, that he represented, as she put it, a "lifeline."

RESEARCH ON ATTACHMENT AND AGGRESSION

Quite apart from content, what distinguishes attachment and psychoanalytic theories is the extensive systematic empirical research generated by the former and the relative lack of it in the latter. Let me turn now to some illustrative examples of the relationship between attachment and aggression.

This can be discussed in a number of different contexts: (1) the child's aggression toward his or her peers, (2) the child's aggression toward his or her caregiver, (3) the caregiver's aggression toward the child, and (4) aggression in adult intimate relationships.

The Child's Aggression toward Peers

The issue of the child's aggression toward his or her peers is especially important insofar as peer relationships in childhood are a relatively robust predictor of later adjustment (e.g., Parker & Asher, 1987). There is a good deal of evidence that a disorganized attachment pattern is a risk factor for aggressive behavior toward peers. Lyons-Ruth (1996) reported that when *combined with the presence* of psychosocial problems in mother, more than 50% of children classified as disorganized in infancy were rated by kindergarten teachers as hostile compared to 5% of children with *neither* of these two risk factors. Shaw, Keenan, Vondra, Delliquadri, and Giovanelli (1997) reported that 60% of children classified as disorganized showed clinically elevated levels of aggression compared to 30% of insecure children and

17% of secure children. Finally, see Jacobvitz and Hazen (1999) for findings on the relationship between infant disorganization and later peer relationships.

There is also a good deal of evidence regarding the relationship between insecure attachment and aggression. Sroufe (1983) and Sroufe, Schork, Motti, Lawroski, and LaFreniere (1984) found that elementary school teachers, using Q-sorts, reported more anger and aggression for insecure than secure children. Observing children in play pairs, Troy and Sroufe (1987) found that avoidant children were more likely to victimize their play partners, whereas anxious–resistant children were more likely to be victims if they were paired with an avoidant child. Secure children were neither victimizers nor victims. Renken, Egeland, Marvinney, Mangelshdof, and Sroufe (1989) found that avoidant boys were rated as more aggressive by elementary school teachers than secure or anxious–resistant boys. Furthermore, avoidant attachment was predictive of conduct problems at age 16 (Aguilar, Sroufe, Egeland, & Carlson, 2000).

The results from the longitudinal National Institute of Child Health and Human Development Study of Early Child Care on 1,060 children found that children who were classified as avoidant at 15 months of age demonstrated more aggressive behavior at 3 years of age than ambivalent or secure children. Aguilar et al. (2000) reported that adolescent antisocial behavior that has an early onset is associated with avoidant attachment at 12 and 18 months. As a final example of the relationship between attachment and aggression, Cassidy and Berlin (1994) and Sroufe et al. (2005b) reported that whereas *ambivalent* children tend to be inhibited and anxiously seek positive peer interaction, avoidant children tend to be aggressive and to repudiate such interactions. In general, avoidant children tend to show externalizing problem behaviors, and ambivalent children tend to show internalizing behaviors.

What might account for the relationship between avoidant attachment and aggressive behavior? As we know, underlying the avoidant pattern is an internal working model characterized by, among other features, the expectation of rejection. One can speculate that the expectation of rejection triggers a "preemptive" hostility, which in turn, makes rejection more likely, thus perpetuating a vicious circle, which serves to confirm the early internal working model.

A study by Dodge, Pettit, Bates, and Valente (1995) in which they found that of a group of adolescent boys who had been physically punished in childhood, only a subsample *who had developed a hostile attributional style* showed a high level of aggressive behavior. Here one aspect of the link between early experiences and later aggression seems relatively clear: Early physical punishment led to the development of a hostile attributional style in some children, which, in turn, lowered their threshold for aggressive behavior. We do not know why only a subsample of the boys who were subjected to early physical punishment developed a hostile attributional style. However, once such a style develops, it is likely to lead to a vicious circle that triggers reactive hostility from others, which, in turn, serves to reinforce the existing hostile attributional style. One can expect that a similar maladaptive cycle is likely to be present in the avoidant pattern–aggressive behavior connection.

The Child's Aggression toward His or Her Caregiver

There is a good deal of research investigating individual differences in aggression toward the caregiver as a function of different attachment patterns. Thus, there is evidence that both avoidant and ambivalent 2-year-old infants show more anger and aggression toward mother than secure infants (Frankel & Bates, 1990; Matas, Arend, & Sroufe, 1978).

One sees this already in 1-year-old ambivalent and avoidant infants in the Strange Situation. However, the patterns of aggressive behavior appear to be different. The ambivalent infant cries bitterly, cannot be comforted, slaps away toys offered, and seems to communicate the message: "How dare you, you have abandoned me. Look what you have done to me." The avoidant infant turns away in a cold and subtle expression of anger, continues playing with his or her toys, and communicates the message: "I don't need you."

Given the lack of any coherent strategy, it is difficult to find any specific communicative meaning expressed in the disorganized infant's bizarre behavior. For these children, aggression toward the caregiver emerges later in development. There is evidence that disorganized attachment in infancy is predictive of controlling behavior toward mother, either punitive or caregiving, at age 6 (Main & Cassidy, 1988; Wartner et al., 1994). Solomon, George, and De Jong (1995) have reported that controlling behavior in doll play is associated with ratings of higher levels of aggression by teachers.

The Caregiver's Aggression toward the Child

Caregiver aggression toward children can be expressed in the indirect form of neglect or in the direct form of physical abuse, with different consequences for attachment status. Finzi, Ram, Har-Even, Shnit, and Weizman

(2001) have shown that neglect is associated with anxious–ambivalent attachment, while physical abuse is associated with avoidant attachment and later aggressive behavior. According to Johnson, Cohen, Chen, Kasen, and Brook (2006), the relative absence of early affection and nurturance is more strongly associated with a wide range of pathology in early adulthood (e.g., borderline personality disorder) than physical and sexual abuse. More generally, there is evidence that harsh child rearing is predictive of later aggressive behavior.

There is a large literature on the effects of parental neglect, maltreatment, and abuse as well as of different forms of child rearing on the development of the child (e.g., Toth, Cicchetti, Macfie, & Emde, 1997; Toth, Manly, & Cicchetti, 1992). A good deal of evidence has been presented that maltreatment in childhood is associated with, among other correlates, aggression as well as both insecure and disorganized attachment patterns. Maltreated children have been found to have rates of insecure attachment as high as 95% as well as elevated levels of disorganized attachment (Cicchetti, Rogosch, & Toth, 2006). In other words, there is a cluster of factors that includes maltreatment, insecure and disorganized attachment, and aggressive behavior.

As Main and Hesse (1990) note, when the caregiver is both the source of danger and anxiety as well as of potential comfort, no coherent strategy is possible. This dilemma is poignantly illustrated in an earlier study in which in response to the noxious stimulus of a puff of air that is emitted whenever the infant monkey approaches its caregiver, the infant clings even more intensely (Harlow, 1960).

The evidence that punishment intensifies rather than attenuates attachment behavior should put to rest the hypothesis that attachment to the caregiver is a simple matter of positive reinforcement (see Chapter 7). That punishment can intensify attachment is consistent with the observation that many maltreated and neglected children in foster care continue to idealize and long for the very caregivers who maltreated and neglected them (R. S. Eagle, 1990, 1993, 1994). According to Fairbairn (1952), such idealization is due to the child taking the badness of the object into himself or herself in order to keep alive the representation of a good object.

Caregiver aggression can also be expressed in the form of what Lieberman (1999) refers to as "negative maternal attributions." In one case she reported, the young single mother interprets the infant's hunger cries as "greed" and makes the baby wait to be fed until she is frantic, which then serves to confirm the mother's attribution of greed to the infant. It is apparent from the material presented that the mother is projecting onto her infant her own condemnatory assessment of her own needs as constituting greed.

Another common source of adult aggression toward the infant that one observes in clinical work is the father's resentment of his spouse's attention to their infant. It is not uncommon to hear in couple therapy that everything was fine until the new baby came along and that after that event, the relationship began to falter. The new father's resentment is often expressed not only in hostility toward his wife, but also toward the infant in a variety of ways, ranging from emotional withdrawal and neglect to physical abuse.

Effect of Witnessing Violence on Children

The above section has dealt with the effects of caregiver aggression on children. However, there is evidence that even if the child is not the direct object of aggression, simply *witnessing* aggression and violence, particularly when they involve the child's attachment figure(s), can have markedly deleterious effects on the child's development.[2] There is much evidence indicating that witnessing domestic violence is associated with increased likelihood of behavior problems and depression (Sternberg et al., 1993); increased incidence of posttraumatic stress disorder (Kilpatrick & Williams, 1997); increased likelihood of domestic violence perpetration or victimization later in life (Whitfield, Anda, Dube, & Felitti, 2003); lower social competence (e.g., Davis & Carlson, 1987); and a variety of other negative outcomes. I have already noted the relationship between the child's experience of his or her caregiver's frightened/frightening behavior and disorganized attachment. Witnessing domestic violence combines the experiences of *both* a frightening adult figure—the perpetrator of the violence—and a frightened figure—the object of the violence. As such, it would be likely to have a powerful negative effect on the child.

Aggression in Adult Intimate Relationships

There is a good deal of evidence that aggression and violence in adult intimate relationships is lawfully related to individual attachment patterns and to the "match" of attachment patterns between partners. With regard to the former, Babcock, Jacobson, Gottman, and Yerington (2000) reported

---

[2] Although far from perfectly correlated, physical abuse of the child and domestic violence—as well as other family stressors—tend to go together.

that violent husbands tend to be more insecurely attached than unhappily married but nonviolent husbands. There is also evidence that violent men in intimate partner violence tend to be more preoccupied and disorganized (Holtzworth-Munroe, Stuart, & Hutchinson, 1997).

With regard to the issue of "match" between attachment patterns, Doumas, Pearson, Elgin, and McKinley (2008) reported that the combination of an avoidant man and anxious woman is associated with both male and female violence. Babcock et al. (2000) found that for male batterers who are preoccupied, the women's withdrawal is a trigger for violence; and for male batterers who are avoidant, the women's withdrawn defensiveness is a trigger for violence. When the avoidant partner turns away or tries to disengage, the preoccupied partner may strike out violently. They note that fear of abandonment is operative in the former and need for control in the latter. However, as Bartholomew and Allison (2006) have reported, a high level of attachment anxiety is especially predictive of intimate partner violence when it is paired with a partner high in attachment avoidance.

The relationship between fear of abandonment and intimate partner violence is especially interesting in the context of attachment theory. It will be recalled that, according to Bowlby (1973), the child's reactions of protest and anger are predictable responses to loss and separation from the attachment figure, the adaptive function of which is to discourage further separation. Note that what is a largely adaptive response of protest and anger in childhood is *maladaptive* in the context of intimate partner violence. What began as an adaptive "situational" response (i.e., to separation) has become transformed into a personality trait, characterized by a chronic fear of potential abandonment, a low threshold for activation of this fear, and a reaction of rage. Whereas protest and anger in a child are generally not dangerous, aggression in an adult with poor impulse control and a poor capacity for mentalization (Fonagy, 1999) can, indeed, be very dangerous and destructive.

A number of additional issues should be noted in a discussion of the relationship between attachment and aggression. Domestic violence is characterized by a pattern that has come to be known as the "cycle of violence," one stage of which is reconciliation and make-up, which serves as a form of intermittent reinforcement for returning to the abusive attachment figure. Another issue has to do with object choice. For many women in a domestic violence situation, the abusive pattern fits the template of an early parental figure who, however abusive and neglectful he or she might have been, also met at least some of her attachment needs. And finally, for some of the women, abuse is equivalent to or a pointer to love. One woman in a group of women involved in domestic violence that Dr. Mindy Puopolo and I ran described her partner's extreme jealousy—which often culminated in violence—with almost a sense of pride and satisfaction because it indicated how much he loved her. The same woman was told by her mother when, as a child, she was physically abused by her father: "He wouldn't do that if he didn't love you."

Although the studies I have noted may be understood as suggesting a straightforward linear relationship between attachment pattern and aggressive behavior, the fact is that the relationship can be quite complex and needs to be contextualized in regard to a number of factors, including age, type of aggression, situational factors, and psychopathology. For example, as noted, whereas avoidant attachment in childhood is associated with externalizing and antisocial behavior, in adulthood and in the context of intimate relationships, it is the combination of a preoccupied individual paired with a partner who is avoidant that is most predictive of violence (Bartholomew & Allison, 2006).

As another example of the importance of context, individuals high in attachment anxiety withhold expressions of anger toward partner when expecting to undergo an anxiety-provoking experience, but show more intense expression of anger when told that they do not have to undergo the experience (Rholes, Simpson, & Orina, 1999). As a final example, individuals diagnosed with borderline personality disorder who show a fearful attachment pattern show a relatively high level of expectation of hostility from others and reactive anger, whereas individuals high in attachment anxiety tend to show higher levels of anger and irritability (Critchfield, Levy, Clarkin, & Kernberg, 2008).

CONCLUDING COMMENTS

The above studies on the relationship between attachment and aggression may suggest that vicissitudes of attachment experiences are the sole source of aggressive behavior. This is, of course, not so. Psychoanalytic theorists and clinicians as well as others identify other sources or aggression, for example, narcissistic injury[3] or aggression fused with sexuality or modeling. However, with few exceptions (e.g., Parens, 1979), the psychoanalytic literature has provided little systematic empirical data on the origin and nature of aggression. In contrast, as we have seen, attachment

---

[3] Abandonment can also be experienced as a narcissistic injury, that is, as a dire threat to self-esteem.

theory has generated a great deal of research on the relationship between attachment and aggression. What seems to emerge from this research is that early attachment experiences that are linked to insecure and disorganized attachment are also conducive to aggression toward peers and toward one's attachment figure, both in childhood and adulthood. Furthermore, common factors that seem to mediate the relationship between attachment and aggression have to do with loss, separation, abandonment, and fears of abandonment—factors that threaten the attachment relationship.

CHAPTER 10

Attachment and Psychopathology

My primary purposes in this chapter are to (1) briefly compare attachment and psychoanalytic theories of psychopathology, (2) highlight some conceptual and methodological issues that emerge from that comparison, and (3) present some illustrative research on the relationship between attachment patterns and psychopathology. (For excellent sources that summarize studies on the relationship between attachment patterns and psychopathology, see DeKlyen & Greenberg, 2008; Dozier et al., 2008; Lyons-Ruth & Jacobvitz, 2008.)

A general basic assumption shared by attachment and psychoanalytic theories is that early experiences, particularly with caregivers, exert powerful influences on development, including the development of psychopathology. Beyond that general commonality, attachment theory and psychoanalytic theories, particularly Freudian and Kleinian theories, present divergent views of the origin and nature of psychopathology. The divergence lessens considerably in regard to contemporary psychoanalytic theories.

CLASSICAL THEORY AND PSYCHOPATHOLOGY

There are at least two aspects to the differences between classical psychoanalytic and attachment theories of psychopathology. One has to do with the content and the other with the method and formal structure of the different theories. With regard to content, both Kleinian and Freudian theories attribute psychopathology to the vicissitudes, anxieties, and conflicts surrounding sexual and aggressive drives (the prototype of which is the Oedipus complex). In contrast, according to attachment theory, psychopathology is mainly attributable to trauma, disruptions, and failures in attachment experiences and the attachment bond.

As for method and formal structure of theories, when one states that early experiences influence later development of personality and psychopathology, one is essentially enunciating an *etiological* theory. It is perhaps surprising to realize that despite its emphasis on early experiences, classical psychoanalytic theory offers a very limited etiological theory. If one examines the corpus of Freud's work, one finds few references to specific early experiences or events associated with specific outcomes.

The specific references one does find are in his early writings—for example, his seduction hypothesis (which, as we know, he essentially relinquished); his speculation that certain early sexual experiences of one kind predispose the individual to phobic symptoms and that sexual experiences of another kind predispose the individual to obsessive symptoms (Freud, 1950[1895], p. 345); and his *fixation* hypothesis to the effect that either overfrustration or overgratification at particular psychosexual stages predisposes the individual to certain character structures (Freud, 1916–1917/1961, p. 340). He also proposed that genetic factors may play a predisposing role in the development of neurosis (his "etiological" or "complemental" series; 1893/1966, 1916–1917/1961, p. 346). None of these early etiological hypotheses, however, plays a major role in psychoanalytic theorizing or in psychoanalytic treatment.

Freud (1920/1955) makes clear that in his view psychoanalysis is a *retrodictive* rather than *predictive* discipline. Bowlby (1969/1982) cites the following passages from Freud to distinguish his approach from Freud's:

> So long as we trace the development from its final outcome backwards, the chain of events appears continuous, and we feel we have gained an insight which is completely satisfactory and even exhaustive. But if we proceed the reverse way, if we start from the premises inferred from the analysis and try to follow these up to the final result, then we no longer get the impression of an inevitable sequence of events which could not have been otherwise determined. We notice at once that there might have been another result, and that we might have been just as well able to understand and explain the latter. The synthesis is thus not so satisfactory as the analysis; in other words, from a knowledge of the premises, we could not have foretold the nature of the result.
>
> Even supposing that we have a complete knowledge of the aetiologocal factors that decide a given result. ... we never know beforehand which of the determining factors will prove the weaker or the stronger.

We only say at the end that those which succeeded must have been the stronger. Hence the chain of causation can always be recognized with certainty if we follow the line of analysis, whereas to predict it along the line of synthesis is impossible. (pp. 167–168)

Thus, according to Freud, psychoanalytic accounts attempt to make sense of developments—for example, neurotic symptoms, inhibitions—that have already occurred rather than try to predict various outcomes. For example, Freud (1925a/1959, p. 55) traces back various manifestations of psychopathology to an inadequate resolution of the Oedipus complex. This can be viewed as an etiological hypothesis in the sense that a failure to resolve Oedipal conflicts is posited to lead to particular outcomes. However, it is a very incomplete etiological hypothesis insofar as it does not identify (or attempt to identify) the factors that influence the degree of adequacy of resolution of Oedipal conflicts. Given the clinical treatment context of much of the psychoanalytic literature and given the assumption that understanding one's past is therapeutic, this retrodictive emphasis makes much sense. However, the result is an impoverished predictive etiological theory.

Thus, that some or many individuals with a history of, say, trauma or conflict do not succumb to neurosis is of little interest to the analyst who is treating the individual who has succumbed. However, to the extent that psychoanalysis is a theory of personality development, including the development of psychopathology, the question of who succumbs to psychopathology and who does not should be of great interest and importance. That it has not been reflects not only the tension between psychoanalysis as treatment and psychoanalysis as theory, but also the near exclusive reliance of psychoanalytic theorizing on *follow-back data* (to be discussed later), that is, the development of etiological theory based largely on data from the clinical situation. This approach simply cannot provide an adequate general etiological account of the development of psychopathology.

CONTEMPORARY PSYCHOANALYTIC THEORIES AND PSYCHOPATHOLOGY

Insofar as they place greater emphasis on environmental events (e.g., maternal failure), contemporary psychoanalytic theories such as self psychology, object relations theory, and relational psychoanalysis are, in principle, more etiologically compatible with an attachment theory etiological perspective.[1]

---

[1] I am not referring here to relative emphasis on early experiences in clinical work, but rather to the content and structure of the theories.

Along with attachment theory, they all share a common emphasis on the critical importance of early relationships and attribute much of psychopathology to failures in these relationships. For example, for Kohut (1984), self defects are attributable to the traumatic lack of parental empathic mirroring; for Fairbairn (1952), "splits in the ego" are due to parental rejection and deprivation; for Winnicott (1965), a "false self" is a response to caregiver impingements; and for Weiss and Sampson (1986), "unconscious pathogenic beliefs" are based on parental communications to the child.

In addition, at least some contemporary theories share with attachment theory an emphasis on the consequences of early negative experiences in the form of maladaptive representations and the persistence of early modes of relating as central aspects of psychopathology. Thus, the approximate counterparts of the attachment theory concepts of attachment patterns and internal working models include Fairbairn's (1952) internalized object relations; Mitchell's (1988) relational configurations; and Kohut's (1984) self–selfobject relations.

ATTACHMENT THEORY AND PSYCHOPATHOLOGY

As noted in Chapter 1, Bowlby's early observation of the pathogenic consequences of maternal deprivation, loss, separation, and threats of separation exerted a strong influence on his development of attachment theory. Although, as also noted, attachment patterns should not be construed as measures of mental illness and mental health,[2] nevertheless an assumption of attachment theory is that secure attachment is a protective factor and insecure attachment a risk factor for psychopathology. The basic rationale underlying intervention programs with infant–mother dyads is the expectation that enhancing the infant's security of attachment will serve as a protective factor against later psychopathology (to be discussed in the next chapter).

Waters et al. (2002) have noted that one of Bowlby's motives in developing attachment theory was to preserve Freud's insight regarding the importance of early experiences in shaping personality. However, the hypothesis that a possible consequence of early negative experiences is a negative developmental trajectory is not uniquely linked to attachment theory (or to psychoanalytic theories). The formulations that are distinctively linked to attachment theory are the assumptions (1) that certain kinds of experiences

---

[2] One should note, however, that indiscriminate attachment as well as failure to develop an attachment bond in children are viewed as attachment disorders (e.g., Zeanah, 1996; Zeanah et al., 2005).

at the hands of caregiver (e.g., rejection of attachment needs) are especially conducive to a negative developmental trajectory and (2) that the negative developmental trajectory is mediated by insecure and disorganized patterns of attachment and their underlying internal models. Also distinctively linked to attachment theory is the generation of a body of research that attempts to test specific hypotheses on the effects of attachment-related experiences on the development of psychopathology.

RESEARCH ON ATTACHMENT PATTERNS AND PSYCHOPATHOLOGY

The research on the relationship between individual differences in attachment patterns and psychopathology has been investigated (1) by examining *concurrent* links between the two, (2) by what one might call *quasi-longitudinal studies* that look at the relationship between infant attachment patterns and psychopathology in early and middle childhood, and (3) by *longitudinal studies* relating early attachment patterns to adult psychopathology. Next I provide some illustrative research in each of these three categories.

Concurrent Studies: Current Attachment Patterns and Current Psychopathology

ATTACHMENT PATTERNS AND EATING DISORDERS

Some examples of concurrent studies include the finding that women who reported eating disorders were most frequently classified as dismissing on the AAI (Cole-Detke & Kobak, 1996; Ward et al., 2001). In contrast, Fonagy et al. (1996) found that eating disorders were most strongly associated with a preoccupied attachment pattern. Clearly, further research is needed to resolve this discrepancy.

ATTACHMENT PATTERNS AND ANXIETY

Rosenstein and Horowitz (1996) reported that 65% of adolescents with clinically elevated scores on the anxiety scale of the Millon Multiaxial Personality Inventory (Millon, 1983), received a preoccupied classification on the AAI. Fonagy et al. (1996) found a similar relationship between anxiety and a preoccupied attachment classification. This finding provides some support for the interpretation of preoccupied attachment in terms of anxiety over fears of abandonment combined with a relative failure of defense.

ATTACHMENT PATTERNS AND BORDERLINE PERSONALITY DISORDER

A number of investigators have reported a significant association between borderline personality disorder and a preoccupied attachment classification (e.g., Barone, 2003; Diamond, Stovall-McClough, Clarkin, & Levy, 2003; Fonagy et al., 1996; Patrick, Hobson, Castle, Howard, & Maughan, 1994; Rosenstein & Horowitz, 1996) as well as unresolved and fearful classifications (Agrawal et al., 2004). Employing the Bartholomew semistructured clinical interview, Lessard and Moretti (1998) found a significant relationship between suicidal ideation and fearful and preoccupied attachment in an adolescent clinical sample. Also, recall the Adam et al. (1996) study which reported that whereas the classification of preoccupied attachment on the AAI was a risk factor for suicide in adolescent hospitalized patients, avoidant attachment was a protective factor.

ATTACHMENT PATTERNS AND DEPRESSION

In view of the fact that according to attachment theory, insecure attachment is a risk factor, it should be associated with psychopathology, including depression. Although there is evidence for this association, the findings are complicated. Internalizing problems, which are linked to depression, have been found to be associated with avoidant attachment (Finnegan, Hodges, & Perry, 1996; Yunger, Corby, & Perry, 2005); ambivalent–preoccupied attachment (Finnegan et al., 1996; Yunger et al., 2005); and disorganized attachment (Graham & Easterbrooks, 2000) in middle childhood.

Employing self-report measures with adults, depression has been found to be associated with preoccupied and fearful attachment (Carnelley, Pietromonaco, & Jaffe, 1994; Hammen, Burger, Daley, & Davila, 1995). In adolescent samples, insecure attachment to parents has been linked to depression (Nada Raja, McGee, & Stanton, 1992). Employing the AAI, one set of investigators has reported a relationship between depression and preoccupied attachment pattern (Cole-Detke & Kobak, 1996; Fonagy et al., 1996: Rosenstein & Horowitz, 1996). However, other investigators have found a closer association between depression and an avoidant pattern of attachment (Patrick et al., 1994). The results have been equally inconsistent with regard to the relationship between unresolved for loss and depression. Thus, Fonagy et al. (1996) found that 72% of depressed inpatients were classified as unresolved, whereas Rosenstein and Horowitz (1996) reported only 18% for an adolescent inpatient sample.

In examining these and other inconsistent findings, Dozier et al. (2008) note the role of different exclusion criteria in at least partly accounting for the inconsistencies. Thus, in the Rosenstein and Horowitz (1996) study,

69% of adolescents who met the diagnostic criteria for major depressive disorder, dysthymia, or schizoaffective disorder were classified as preoccupied, whereas only 25% of the comorbid group (affective disorder plus conduct disorder) were classified as preoccupied, with most of them being classified as dismissing. Furthermore, 75% of the affective disorder group also had personality disorder diagnoses, most of whom were classified as preoccupied. In short, because of such factors as comorbidity and the presence of personality disorders, one can draw no clear-cut conclusions regarding the relationship between depression and attachment patterns.

One should add another consideration. According to Blatt (2004), there are at least two forms of depression: anaclitic depression, which has more to do with loss and rejection in interpersonal relations; and introjective depression, which has more to do with issues of failure and not living up to one's ideals. One could hypothesize that anaclitic depression would be associated with preoccupied attachment and unresolved for loss, whereas introjective depression would be more closely associated with avoidant attachment.

ATTACHMENT PATTERNS AND ALEXITHYMIA

Based on self-report measures of attachment patterns, Troisi, D'Argenio, Peracchio, and Petti (2001) found that among young men with clinically significant mood symptoms, preoccupied and fearful attachment was more strongly associated with alexithymia than a secure or dismissive pattern.

ATTACHMENT PATTERNS AND SOMATOFORM DISORDERS

In an AAI study on patients with an *International Classification of Diseases* diagnosis of somatoform disorders compared with 20 healthy control subjects, Waller, Scheidt, and Hartmann (2004) reported a higher incidence of insecure attachment in the somatoform group than in the control group. Further, in the somatoform group, dismissing attachment was twice as prevalent as preoccupied attachment. The overrepresentation of somatization in the dismissive group is congruent with O'Shea-Lauber's (2000) similar finding employing self-report measure of attachment as well as with the evidence that a "repressive style" is associated with susceptibility to certain physical symptoms (e.g., Schwartz, 1990).

ATTACHMENT PATTERNS AND GENERAL PSYCHOPATHOLOGY

A number of studies have been carried out examining the incidence of a psychopathology diagnosis in individuals with different attachment patterns.

Ward, Leer, and Polan (2006) reported that 63% of dismissing women, 100% of preoccupied women, and 68% of women with unresolved AAI narratives received Structured Clinical Interview for DSM-III-R diagnoses compared to 32% of women with secure–autonomous AAI narratives. They also found that a dismissing classification was associated with Axis I diagnoses and that preoccupied classification was associated with affective disorders.

ATTACHMENT PATTERNS AND DISSOCIATIVE SYMPTOMS

West, Adam, Spreng, and Rose (2001) found that "Unresolved" or "Cannot Classify" on the AAI was more frequent among adolescent inpatients with higher dissociation scores. The association between unresolved trauma and dissociative symptomatology was also reported by Riggs et al. (2007). And finally Stovall-McClough and Cloitre (2006) found a modest but statistically significant association between unresolved on the AAI and self-report of dissociative symptoms.

FOLLOW-BACK VERSUS FOLLOW-UP DESIGNS

With the exception of the Ward et al. (2006) study, all the above studies, which are representative of concurrent studies in the literature, employ a "follow-back" design.[3] That is, in such research one typically takes a sample of individuals who are diagnosed with psychopathology and then looks at the percentage of them who are insecurely attached compared to the percentage of a control group. However, what if one began with a large random sample of insecurely attached individuals and then looked at how many of them showed diagnosable psychopathology? It is very likely that in this "follow-up" procedure, the relationship between attachment insecurity and psychopathology would be much weaker compared to a "follow-back" procedure.

An etiological theory based mainly on the "follow-back" method will be incomplete and misleading as far as the strength of the relationship between attachment patterns and psychopathology is concerned. At the very least, the "follow-up" findings would likely indicate that the relationship between insecure attachment and psychopathology is a complex one that is mediated by other factors and would point to the need for future

---

[3]The Ward et al. (2006) study employed a follow-up design in the sense that it began with a sample of insecurely and securely attached women and then asked how many of these women received a diagnosis of psychopathology. However, the sample was a high-risk rather than a random one.

research on the identification of these other factors and of the processes involved.

As a concrete example, consider the relationship between insecure attachment and borderline pathology. If one takes a sample of borderline patients, a large number of them will be insecurely attached, likely fearful, enmeshed/preoccupied and unresolved (Agrawal et al., 2004). Such studies have justifiably identified insecure attachment as a risk factor for borderline pathology. However, that is only part of the story. For these studies are almost always characterized by the use of *follow-back* rather than follow-up or longitudinal data. That is to say, a sample of borderline patients are identified, and one then "looks back" to see how many are insecurely versus securely attached. The limitations of this approach are indicated by the following hypothetical example.

Let us say that we start with a large sample of 1,000 insecurely attached individuals and let us say that 10% of the sample is shown to have borderline pathology. This certainly would suggest some relationship between insecure attachment and borderline pathology insofar as it is unlikely that 10% of a securely attached sample would show borderline pathology (one's control group would, of course, consist of securely attached individuals). However, something very important about the nature of strength of relationship between insecure attachment and borderline pathology would be reflected in the fact that 90% of the insecurely attached sample does not show borderline pathology.

Furthermore, the 100 individuals who show borderline pathology will be far more likely to be seen by mental health practitioners than the 900 insecurely attached individuals who do not show borderline pathology. Indeed, imagine that all of the 100 borderline individuals are seen at a particular mental health center and imagine further that a research paper from that center reports that 100% of borderline patients seen during a particular period were all insecurely attached. It would be very tempting on this basis to overestimate the strength of the relationship between insecure attachment and borderline pathology.

The problems I have noted are not limited to the relationship between attachment patterns and psychopathology, but are present in all etiological theories that are mainly based on clinical follow-back data from individuals who show psychopathology. This is as true of, say, cognitive behavioral as of psychoanalytic etiological theories. With regard to the former, even if all depressed patients show irrational beliefs of a certain kind, we do not know what percentage of individuals with these irrational beliefs become depressed.

Quasi-Longitudinal Studies: Early Attachment Patterns and Childhood Psychopathology

As we have seen in Chapter 3, there is evidence that early attachment patterns influence cognitive and social functioning in later childhood. The question addressed here, however, is whether early attachment patterns are predictive of psychopathology in later childhood. There is relatively clear evidence that early disorganized attachment is predictive, among other outcomes, of poorer academic performance (e.g., Moss, St. Laurent, & Parent, 1999), and teacher reports of dissociation in grades 1, 2, and 3 (Carlson, 1998), as well as at age 17½ (Carlson, 1998), and age 19 (Ogawa et al., 1997). Lewis, Feiring, McGuffog, and Jaskir (1984) reported that 40% of insecure boys, as compared to 6% of secure boys, scored above the 90th percentile on the Child Behavioral Checklist (CBCL) Total Problem Score. However, attachment status was no longer predictive at age 13.

As DeKlyen and Greenberg (2008) have pointed out, for the most part, early attachment as a main effect has not been very predictive of childhood psychopathology. However, as shown in the above Lyons-Ruth et al. (1996) study, early attachment status becomes more predictive in interaction with other variables. And one of the main variables that adds predictive value is high- versus low-risk environment. As Dekleyen and Greenberg (2008) note, even a large sample of the National Institute of Child Health and Human Development study of early child care (Belsky & Fearon, 2002) did not yield a main effect, but "was only predictive of problem behavior within the context of high-risk environment" (p. 645). They conclude that "children in high social-risk environments who exhibited early insecurity [and, one could add, early disorganized attachment] are significantly more likely to have poor peer relations and more symptoms of aggression, depression, and general maladjustment later than are children with early security" (p. 645).

Longitudinal Studies: Early Attachment Patterns and Adult Psychopathology

A number of major longitudinal studies have been done on early attachment and later development (Grossmann, Grossmann, & Waters, 2005). However, although these studies have covered a wide range of outcomes, very little work has been done on the relationship between early attachment patterns and adult psychopathology. Indeed, the index of the Grossmann et al. (2005) volume contains one single-page entry on "psychopathology."

Dozier et al. (2008) write that "the evidence specifically linking infant's attachment behavioral strategies to psychopathology in adulthood is limited to a few longitudinal studies" (p. 719). The few longitudinal studies that have been carried out show the following:

1. Both avoidant and disorganization classifications in infancy are predictive of dissociation in adolescence and young adulthood (Carlson, 1998; Dutra & Lyons-Ruth, 2005; Ogawa et al., 1997).
2. Infants with resistant attachment were significantly more likely to be diagnosed with anxiety disorders at age 17 than secure or avoidant infants (Bosquet & Egeland, 2006; Warren, Huston, Egeland, & Sroufe, 1997).

After surveying the literature on the relationship between early attachment patterns and adult psychopathology, Dozier et al. (2008) conclude: "At this point, the only clear connection between infant attachment and adult psychopathology are between disorganized attachment and dissociative symptoms in adolescence and early adulthood ... and between resistant attachment and anxiety disorders in adolescence" (p. 736). This conclusion should not be surprising given the complex nature of development and the fact that attachment pattern is only one of many variables that influence an individual's developmental trajectory. I would reiterate the generalization that early attachment patterns are likely to be predictive of later psychopathology (as well as other aspects of development) not as main effects, but in interaction with other variables (e.g., high-risk vs. low-risk environments).

The research findings of longitudinal studies should serve to place realistic restraints on the temptation to overemphasize the role of early attachment patterns on the individual's susceptibility to psychopathology in adulthood. Although the role of individual differences in the development of psychopathology is of great interest to attachment theory, they are likely to represent one set of factors—albeit an important set—that are predictive of psychopathology.

Even if early attachment patterns did reliably predict later psychopathology, it would be a mistake to conclude that there is necessarily a direct causal link between attachment pattern at time 1 (say, at 1 year or 18 months of age) and "outcome" at time N. It is very likely that success in predicting from time 1 to time N is at least partly due to the fact that the factors that were operating in the development of a particular attachment pattern at time 1 continued to be operative in different age-related forms at times 2, 3, 4, and so on. If this is so, it is not attachment pattern at time 1, but cumulative factors that contribute to attachment patterns at times 2, 3, 4, and so on that are predictive of outcome at time N.

Another important consideration that one must keep in mind in relating early attachment patterns (or any set of early experiences) to later psychopathology is the route traversed from one to the others. The assumption of a linear etiological model of a single train track on which one gets from A to B was, for Bowlby, a problematic feature of psychoanalytic theorizing. In contrast to this "single-track" model, a more realistic etiological model proposed by attachment theory is that of a train track that starts at point A and switches off at various "choice points" to point C, and so on, some of which go to point B and others of which go to other destinations. It is ironic that some accounts of attachment theorists of the trajectory from early attachment pattern to later development seem more suggestive of a single track rather than a multiple-track model.

The above issues are likely to be relevant not only in the context of the relationship between early attachment and later psychopathology, but also with regard to virtually any model of the relationship between early experiences and later development outcomes. Rutter, Quinton, and Hill's (1990) classic study of the developmental trajectory of girls raised in orphanages nicely illustrates a multiple-track choice points model. A factor as seemingly mundane as doing well at school served as a "choice point" that then increased the likelihood of a longer period of education, which then further influenced such factors as the nature of the girl's peer group, the kind of employment they obtained, the likelihood of finding a stable and supportive mate, timing of pregnancy, and so on. Those girls who did not do well at school showed a different trajectory, characterized by a lower level of education, a less wholesome peer group, fewer employment opportunities, poorer choice of mate, earlier pregnancy, and so on.

Let us assume for the sake of argument that all the girls in Rutter's sample were insecurely attached in infancy. How would one account for their different developmental trajectories? One possibility is that for the subsample of girls with a more positive trajectory, positive later infancy experiences led to a shift from insecure to secure attachment, which then influenced positive school performance and the subsequent cascade of positive "choice points."

This model is given credence, by the evidence noted in Chapter 3, that changes in the environment lead to changes in attachment patterns (although the usual finding is a shift from secure to insecure as a function of environmental disruptions such as loss and illness. According to this model, attachment pattern remains a critical factor in predicting developmental outcomes. However, it would not be early attachment patterns, but the attachment pattern closest in time to the outcome being assessed that would be most predictive. Note that to test this model, one would need to obtain measures of attachment patterns at different periods in the individual's life. As noted in Chapter 4, this task is made more difficult by the unavailability of reliable measures of attachment patterns in the period between infancy and adulthood.

Another possibility is that the girls in the Rutter, Quinton, and Hill (1990) study were and remained insecurely attached and that other factors such as academic talent, persistence, likeability, and so on were mainly responsible for their school performance, which then paved the way for either a relatively positive or negative trajectory. According to this model, other factors can override insecure attachment patterns in influencing development. This model is likely to have a good deal of validity insofar as there are undoubtedly many individuals who were insecurely attached as infants and remain insecurely attached as adults, but nevertheless show a relatively positive life course.

This latter model is consistent with a conception of insecure attachment as a risk factor that can be overridden by other factors. The contribution of a risk factor to psychopathology is always a product of its interaction with other factors. Insecure attachment interacting with one set of factors may result in psychopathology, whereas insecure attachment interacting with a different set of factors may not. This argument also holds for secure attachment. Although secure attachment may serve as a protective factor, under certain circumstances, the protective role of secure attachment may be overridden by other factors, with the development of psychopathology as a consequence.

To complicate matters further, although I have been referring to psychopathology as a global term, the contribution of attachment patterns to the development of psychopathology is likely to be a function of type of pathology. For example, attachment patterns and dynamics have been found to be associated with borderline conditions (e.g., Agrawal et al., 2004; Critchfield et al., 2008), whereas there is less evidence on the relationship between attachment patterns and say, obsessive-compulsive disorders or schizophrenia. This may be due to the relative lack of research in these areas or to the fact that attachment patterns may be less relevant to understanding the etiology of the latter set of disorders.

AVOIDANT VERSUS PREOCCUPIED ATTACHMENT

Different insecure attachment patterns may play different roles in psychopathology. As we have seen in Chapter 3, disorganized attachment in infancy and its counterpart of unresolved in adulthood are especially predictive of psychopathology. As noted earlier, Adam et al. (1996) found that among hospitalized borderline adolescents, being avoidantly attached on the AAI was a protective factor against suicide attempts, whereas being preoccupied plus unresolved were risk factors. In other words, an attachment pattern that is a risk factor for one set of outcomes can be a protective factor in regard to another set of outcomes.

It helps to understand this finding (as well as other related findings) if one thinks of avoidant and preoccupied attachment patterns from the perspective of the psychoanalytic concept of defense. Insofar as an avoidant attachment pattern is associated with relatively intact defense, an avoidantly attached individual is more able to ward off conscious dysphoric feelings such as anxiety and guilt as well as thoughts that are likely to trigger such feelings. In contrast, insofar as preoccupied attachment is associated with a relative failure of defense, this individual will be more likely to consciously experience thoughts and feelings that trigger anxiety and other dysphoric affect.

Hence, it is not surprising that avoidant attachment is a protective factor and preoccupied attachment a risk factor for suicide attempts. This is also congruent with the association between preoccupied attachment and borderline conditions and the general finding that on a wide range of correlates, it is more difficult to distinguish avoidant from secure than preoccupied from secure.

DIMENSIONS VERSUS CATEGORIES

A number of issues pertain to the relationship between attachment and psychopathology that merit further research and conceptual clarification. One such issue has to do with what one might call intensity of attachment pattern. Being mildly or moderately avoidant or preoccupied is likely to have a different adaptive significance than being extremely avoidant or preoccupied. Yet, I do not know of any studies directly investigating this question. One obstacle to such an investigation, at least when the AAI is used to assess attachment patterns, is that it is designed to yield categorical classifications rather than dimensional ratings—although it would seem possible to carry out the latter. As for the self-report questionnaire method, the ECR questionnaire (Brennan, Clark, & Shaver, 1998) is already constructed to yield dimensional ratings on anxiety and avoidance and easily lends itself to studies on "intensity" on each dimension (and their interaction) and psychopathology.

CONCLUDING COMMENTS

As the above brief survey makes clear, apart from content, a major difference between attachment and psychoanalytic theories of psychopathology is the degree to which attachment has generated a body of systematic research, including longitudinal studies. Contrastingly, with rare exceptions (e.g., Vaillant, 1971, 1975, 1976), psychoanalytic theories of psychopathology are based largely on clinical experiences, individual case studies, and clinical vignettes, all derived from the therapeutic situation. The inevitable consequences of this approach include an excessive reliance on follow-back data and, therefore, an incomplete and potentially misleading theory of psychopathology. I want to note that in its current form, attachment theory—qua theory—is not necessarily a superior theory of psychopathology. Rather, insofar as it employs more reliable and valid methods of generating data, it is increasingly likely to develop a more complete and defensible theory of psychopathology.

CHAPTER 11

Implications of Attachment Research and Theory for Clinical Interventions

Attachment theory and research no doubt contribute in important ways to our clinical and theoretical understanding of personality and psychological functioning. The main issue I address in this chapter, however, is the implications of attachment theory and research for clinical interventions. Further, in discussing the implications of attachment theory and research for clinical interventions, I distinguish between interventions with infant–mother dyads and interventions in the form of individual psychotherapy with adults, the latter comprising individual psychotherapy with adults and work with couples. I argue that whereas attachment theory and research have relatively direct implications for the former, this is far less clear with regard to the latter.

IS THERE AN ATTACHMENT-BASED PSYCHOTHERAPY?

Levy, Beeney, and Temes (2011) write that "Fonagy and Bateman's mentalization-based therapy (MBT) is unambiguously based on attachment theory, ... whereas the transference-focused psychotherapy of Levy et al. ... may be conceived as an implicit attachment theory based treatment" (p. 55). The links between mentalization-based therapy and attachment theory, however, are indirect and are more, so to speak, historical than

157

conceptual. As we have seen in Chapter 4, Fonagy and his colleagues (1995) found that level of reflective function accounts for a great portion of the variance in attachment classifications on the AAI. They also found that mother's reflective capacity on the AAI is a robust predictor of the infant's attachment status (Fonagy et al., 1991). However, as Bateman and Fonagy (2006) note, enhancing the individual's ability to reflect on his or her own mental states and those of others, a central feature of MBT, is also a central component of a number of psychotherapeutic approaches, including a classic psychoanalytic approach (i.e., enhancing the observing function of the ego). One can also add Weiss and Sampson's (1986) control–mastery theory (reflecting on one's "unconscious pathogenic beliefs"), and cognitive-behavioral theory (reflecting on one's implicit thoughts and irrational beliefs).

This is not to suggest that there are no differences among these concepts; indeed, there are. Thus, whereas the observing function of the ego pertains mainly to the intrapsychic, mentalization and reflective function also include a focus on mental states of the other. I am suggesting, as do Bateman and Fonagy (2006), that the concepts of mentalization and reflective function are not uniquely linked to attachment theory.

I think the link between transference-focused psychotherapy (TFP) and attachment theory is even more tenuous. Kernberg, Yeomans, Clarkin, and Levy (2008) have made it clear that TFP is based on Kernberg's version of object relations theory, in particular his hypothesis that splitting is a central feature of borderline personality disorder. Also, analysis of the transference has been a core aspect of psychoanalytic treatment since Freud and has been referred to as the "common ground" (Wallerstein, 1990) of psychoanalytic treatment approaches. That a shift from insecure to secure attachment has been employed as an outcome criterion in some TFP research does not indicate that it is an "implicit attachment-based treatment."

One of the issues that arises with regard to so-called attachment-based psychotherapy is that it is often difficult to distinguish between what are essentially rewordings in the language of attachment theory of existing formulations and contributions that are distinctively derived from attachment theory—that is, that, so to speak, require attachment theory in order to be articulated.

In contrast to the rather direct implications of attachment theory and research for therapeutic work with infant–mother dyads, the direct relevance of attachment theory for individual psychotherapy with adults is far less obvious. Despite the outpouring of books and journal articles on attachment theory and psychotherapy—it has become a virtual industry—the fact is that there is no particular or distinctive form of psychotherapy that one can legitimately call attachment therapy in the same way that one can refer to, say, cognitive-behavioral therapy (CBT) or psychoanalytic therapy. Although attachment theory may have important implications for clinical interventions, it does not constitute a therapeutic approach. Nor is it a theory of psychotherapy in the same way that cognitive-behavioral theory or aspects of psychoanalytic theory constitute therapeutic approaches of, respectively, CBT and psychoanalytic or psychodynamic therapy.

Consider two books purporting to present an attachment-based therapeutic approach. In one of them, in a chapter titled "Attachment-Based Psychotherapy," under a heading labeled "Treatment Technique," Brisch (2012) offers the following suggestions in regard to adult psychotherapy:

- In his caregiving behavior, the therapist must allow the help-seeking patient to speak to him via his activated attachment system and make himself emotionally available to the patient. This includes budgeting sufficient time and space.
- The therapist must function as a reliable secure base from which the patient can safely work through his problems.
- Taking the various attachment patterns into consideration, the therapist must be flexible in the way he handles closeness and distance with the patient, both in their interactions and in the establishment of the therapeutic setting.
- The therapist should encourage the patient to think about what attachment strategies he is presently using in his interactions with his important attachment figures.
- The therapist must urge the patient to examine the therapeutic relationship in detail. The therapist himself must do so, as well, because this is where all the perceptions of relationships conditioned by one's representations of one's parents and oneself are reflected.
- The patient should be cautiously encouraged to compare his current perceptions and feelings with those experienced in childhood.
- It should be made clear to the patient that his painful experiences with attachment and relationships, and the distorted representations of self and object that arose from these experiences, are probably inappropriate for dealing with current important relationships: In other words, they are outdated.
- In his careful dissolution of the therapeutic bond, the therapist serves as a model for dealing with separation. Separation is left to the patient's initiative, as a forced separation initiated by the therapist could be experienced as rejection. The patient should be encouraged to verbalize his separation anxieties and his questions about being on his own without the therapist—perhaps even to do some experimenting. Physical separation is not the same as loss of the "secure base." Should the patient need help at a later date, he would still be able to rely on the therapist.

- A therapist who offers more closeness than the patient can handle (and which is therefore experienced as a threat) may trigger a premature desire for separation and/or more distance in the therapeutic relationship in patients with an avoidant pattern of attachment. (pp. 102–103)

Although Brisch's suggestions are couched in the language of attachment theory, most, if not all of them, could be made in a variety of therapeutic approaches that make no reference to attachment theory. The critical question is whether attachment theory is necessary as an underpinning for these "treatment techniques."

Consider also Wallin's (2007) *Attachment in Psychotherapy*. Although similar to Brisch, Wallin invokes attachment theory in his descriptions of his therapeutic approach, and many of the suggestions made have little to do with attachment theory. For example, Wallin devotes much attention to the usefulness of meditation and mindfulness in psychotherapy. Although that may be an interesting topic and worthy of discussion, its relevance to attachment theory is not clear. As another example, Wallin reconsiders psychoanalytic concepts such as transference, countertransference, resistance, neutrality, and self-disclosure from the perspective of relational and intersubjective psychoanalytic theories. Again, although interesting and worthy of discussion, its relevance to attachment theory is not at all clear.

Attachment theory *is* relevant to Wallin's discussion of different attachment patterns. However, its relevance to attachment theory has to do with the importance of taking account of the patient's particular attachment pattern in carrying out treatment rather than with identifying an attachment-based therapeutic approach. Moreover, certain aspects of Wallin's discussion of the role of the patient's attachment pattern can be somewhat misleading. For example, he writes that "preoccupied patients can be seen to fall on a diagnostic continuum with hysterics at one end and borderlines at the other" (p. 224). But the preoccupied attachment is not a diagnostic category or a form of psychopathology. It is within the normal range of distribution of attachment patterns.

Similarly for dismissive attachment, Wallin's description of "avoidant or dismissive [patients as] usually (more or less) 'disembodied'" and as being "gripped by powerful 'reflexes' that constrain their actions and divert attention from their feelings and sensations" (p. 79) renders dismissive attachment as a form of psychopathology. Also, there is little empirical support for these speculative characterizations. One should keep in mind that Wallin is describing patients in treatment who happen to have dismissive or preoccupied attachment patterns rather than the approximately 35–45% of the population who have been classified as avoidant or preoccupied. One should also keep in mind that there are undoubtedly patients in treatment who are classified as securely attached. For these patients, a description of their attachment pattern would not capture the nature of their distress and their reasons for being in treatment. This is also likely to be the case for those patients with insecure patterns of attachment.

I want to make it clear that the books by Brisch and Wallin are quite useful and very much worth reading. My main concern is whether they present an attachment-based therapeutic approach. I have spent all this time on the question of whether there is such a thing as attachment-based psychotherapy because I do not believe that it advances our understanding to essentially relabel a range of concepts and interventions—some familiar and embedded in particular theoretical contexts—as attachment-based owing to the current popularity of attachment theory. I also think that we do not further the development of attachment theory by an excessively loose and relatively indiscriminate rendering of its concepts.

The focus of Bowlby's trilogy is not on psychotherapy—there is relatively little on that topic—but on articulating the basic tenets of attachment theory. Much of what Bowlby does have to say about the implications of attachment theory for adult psychotherapy appears much later and is summarized in Chapter 8 of his 1988 *A Secure Base*. However, even here Bowlby does not formulate an attachment-based therapeutic approach. Helping the patient become aware of and free himself or herself from early maladaptive representations is one goal of treatment identified by Bowlby. However, this goal is central to other therapeutic approaches, including the emphasis of the control-mastery approach on helping the patient become aware of and reflect upon "unconscious pathogenic beliefs" (Weiss & Sampson, 1986); or the emphasis of Freudian and Kleinian analysts on helping the patient free himself or herself from being unduly influenced by early sexual and aggressive fantasies. Also, Klein's (1945) concept of reparation implies recognition of both one's own mental states (e.g., a destructive wish) and the other's mental states (e.g., hurt and suffering). Although attachment theory points to a particular set of maladaptive representations, I think it is a stretch to refer to an attachment-based psychotherapy approach.

I fully agree with this response by Obegi and Berant (2009) to the question "Is there such a thing as 'attachment therapy' for adults?": "There is no school of therapy for adults called 'attachment therapy.' Unlike . . . Sigmund Freud or Aaron Beck[,] John Bowlby did not detail, beyond a rough outline, a therapeutic approach to complement his comprehensive theory" (p. 2). Obegi and Berant go on to distinguish between "attachment-formed" and "attachment-based" psychotherapy. Exemplars of attachment-formed psychotherapy, according to them, include interpersonal therapy (e.g.,

Klerman, Weissman, Rounsaville, & Chevron, 1984); cognitive-analytic therapy (Ryle, 1990); accelerated experiential-dynamic psychotherapy (Fosha, 2000); and, among others, the therapeutic approaches of Byng-Hall (1998), Slade (2008), and Wallin (2007).

As for "attachment-based psychotherapy," Obegi and Berant's (2009) exemplars include Marvin et al.'s (2002) Circle of Security program with infant–mother dyads as well as other infant–mother interventions; emotion-focused therapy (EFT) for couples (Johnson, 2008); brief attachment-based therapy (Holmes, 2001); attachment-based psychoanalytic psychotherapy (White, 2004); and an attachment-guided approach developed by Brisch (2002, p. 3). As will be discussed later in the chapter, interventions with infant–mother dyads are, indeed, closely linked to attachment theory and research. However, one would want to take a close look at other exemplars of "attachment-based" psychotherapy to determine to what degree and in what specific ways they are "attachment-based." My examination of Brisch's (2012) and Wallin's (2007) therapeutic approaches, which are presumably "attachment-guided" or attachment-derived, feeds my skepticism regarding the appellation "attachment-based" applied to the other approaches noted. A careful examination of these other approaches is warranted before one addresses the question of the degree to which they are "attachment-based."

In general, I think Slade (1999) has it right when she observes that "an understanding of the nature of dynamics of attachment *informs* rather than *defines* intervention and clinical thinking" (p. 577). In my view, following Slade, rather than constituting a new therapeutic approach or pointing to new specific interventions, attachment theory informs psychotherapy by alerting and sensitizing the therapist to certain central aspects of the patient's life.

In particular, attachment theory directs the therapist's attention to the patient's implicit expectations regarding the availability of the attachment figure, his or her self-representations and representations of the attachment figure, how these expectations and representations are expressed in the therapeutic situation, and the patient's ways of meeting his or her attachment needs. In short, an attachment theory perspective directs the therapist's attention to exploration of the patient's internal working model or what Main and Hesse (1995) refer to, in the context of the AAI, as the individual's "state of mind with respect to attachment" (p. 68).

Although Freudian and Kleinian theories may have neglected this area of the patient's psychological life, it is attended to and investigated in many, if not most, contemporary therapeutic approaches. For example, Weiss and Sampson's (1986) concept of "unconscious pathogenic beliefs," Fairbairn's

(1952) internalized object relations, Kohut's (1984) self-selfobject relation-ships, Mitchell's (1988) "relational configurations," and Schachter's (2002) "habitual relationship pattern," all bear a family resemblance to the con-cept of internal working model, in particular, its emphasis on interactional representations.

FUNCTION OF THE THERAPIST
FROM AN ATTACHMENT THEORY PERSPECTIVE

Bowlby (1988) wrote that one of the main functions of a therapist "is to provide the patient with a secure base from which he can explore the vari-ous unhappy and painful aspects of his life, past and present, many of which he finds it difficult or perhaps impossible to think about and recon-sider without a trusted companion to provide support, encouragement, sympathy, and, on occasion, guidance" (p. 138). There are two related assumptions implicit in the above passage. One is that the therapist serves as an attachment figure for the patient, an assumption that is supported by empirical evidence (Mallinckrodt, Porter, & Kivligham, 2005; Parish & Eagle, 2003). The other implicit assumption is that a central function of the therapist is to serve as a secure base for the patient. Bowlby, was, of course, aware that this is often not the case. He writes that "the patient will import [into the therapeutic relationship] all those perceptions, constructions, and expectations of how an attachment figure is likely to feel and behave towards him that his working model of parents and self dictate" (p. 138). For example, one would expect that the insecurely attached patient will, early in the treatment, experience the therapist in accord with the expecta-tions and representations that constitute an insecure attachment pattern; that is, this patient will not be especially able to experience the therapist as a secure base. Were the patient able, right from the start, to experience the therapist as a secure base—or safe haven—that much less therapeutic work would need to be done.

Hence, as Bowlby (1988) also notes, much of the therapeutic work will consist in encouraging the patient to become aware of and examine his or her representational models, their origins in his or her interactions with parents, and how they influence his or her interactions with the thera-pist and with current significant figures outside the therapeutic situation. Finally, from an attachment theory perspective, the goal of treatment is the "restructuring of ... [his or her representational models] in the light of the new understanding he acquires and new experiences he has in the therapeu-tic relationship" (p. 138).

Bowlby (1988) also states with regard to the therapist's function that "A therapist applying attachment theory sees his role as being one of providing the conditions in which his patient can explore his representational models of himself and his attachment figures with a view to reappraising and restructuring them in the light of the new understanding he acquires and the new experiences he has in the therapeutic relationship" (p. 138). He also writes that "A particular relationship that the therapist encourages the patient to examine ... is the relationship between the two of them. Into this the patient will import all those perceptions, constructions, and expectations of how an attachment figure is likely to feel and behave towards him that his working models of parents and self dictate" (p. 138). This description of the therapeutic process and of a central therapeutic goal, it will be noted, is similar to the psychoanalytic emphasis on the analysis of the transference. For both attachment theory and psychoanalysis, the expectation is that this process will eventuate in more realistic representations of the analyst and of significant figures in the patient's life.

One can see from the above passages that Bowlby places equal emphasis on the interpretive (i.e., "the new understanding") and "new experiences" in the therapeutic relationship. From an attachment theory perspective, just as is the case in the child's experiences with his or her attachment figure, one would expect that repeated experiences of the therapist as a safe haven in times of distress help establish the therapist as a secure base from which to explore. In this regard, Bowlby's view is similar to contemporary psychoanalytic views. Thus, Weiss and Sampson (1986) refer to tests the therapist must pass if the patient is to feel sufficiently safe to explore anxiety-laden material. Fairbairn (1952) writes about the importance of the therapist being experienced as a "good" object. And Kohut (1984) stresses the importance of the empathic bond between patient and therapist, which rests on the therapist's capacity to deal adequately with inevitable "optimal failures" on his or her part.

Bowlby (1988) states that "readers will be aware that the principles set out have a great deal in common with the principles described by other analytically trained psychotherapists who regard conflicts arising within interpersonal relationships as the key to an understanding of their patient's problems, who focus on the transference and who also give some weight, albeit of varying degree, to a patient's earlier experience with his parents" (p. 139). Bowlby also writes that "in this account of therapeutic principles, therapists will recognize much that has long been familiar, though often under a different name" (p. 151). He refers to Fairbairn, Winnicott, Guntrip, Sullivan, Fromm-Reichmann, Gill, Kohut, Casement, Pine, Strupp, Binder, Malan, and Horowitz as examples of therapists whose approach to psychotherapy shares much in common with the approach of attachment theory.

Bowlby could also have included others, including Stolorow and his colleagues and Freud. Similar to Bowlby, but employing different language, Stolorow, Atwood, and Orange (2002) conceptualize the therapist's role as helping the individual expand his or her "regions of experience" and "horizons of awareness" that have been restricted by parental prohibitions and invalidation of the child's experiences. As for Freud (1926a/1959), he discusses the role of anxiety related to the "danger situations" (p. 129) (which includes loss of the object and of the object's love) in keeping the individual from thinking thoughts and experiencing feelings that have been prohibited by parents. After all, what is repression of thoughts and feelings if not the result of internalized parental prohibitions? And does not the clinical work in classical psychoanalysis designed to lift repression entail the sanctioning of thinking forbidden thoughts and experiencing forbidden feelings?

Bowlby (1988) does identify one "aspect of therapy in which the work of a therapist who adopts attachment theory is likely to differ most from one who adopts certain of the traditional theories of personality development and psychopathology" (p. 141). And that aspect, according to Bowlby, is the difference between viewing the patient's constructions and construals "as the not unreasonable products of what the patient has actually experienced in the past, or has repeatedly been told" (p. 141) versus viewing them "as the irrational offspring of autonomous and unconscious fantasy" (p. 142).

Bowlby has in mind here what he believes to be the overemphasis of Kleinian and Freudian theories on unconscious fantasy and their relative neglect of actual events. However, Bowlby draws too sharp a dichotomy here. With regard to Kleinian theory, as we have seen in Chapter 5, Klein does leave some room for the role of actual events in understanding the patient's experiences. As for Freudian theory, Freud's (1926a/1959) formulation of the child's anxieties in relation to the "danger situations" (p. 129) of loss of the object and loss of the object's love can serve as a model of the interaction among actual events, immature cognition, and fantasy. That is, the child's anxieties are linked to the actual events of parental disapproval and punishment. However, they also entail a mixture of immature cognition and fantasy. Although parental disapproval and punishment may be experienced by the child as loss of the object and of the object's love, this is obviously not generally the parental intention. So, the child's anxieties may well be a reaction to actual events, but a reaction that may be much influenced by fantasies that are fed by the child's immature cognitions—for example, equating parental disapproval with loss of the object.

Another difference between attachment-related and traditional theories of psychotherapy delineated by Bowlby has to do with the role of interpretation. Bowlby (1988) writes that "among the points of difference [between traditional and attachment theorists] is the emphasis placed on the therapist's role as a companion for his patient in the latter's exploration of himself and his experiences, and less on the therapist interpreting things to the patient. Whilst some traditional therapists might be described as adopting the stance 'I know, I'll tell you', the stance I advocate is one of 'You know, you tell me' " (p. 151).

Because Bowlby seems to assume that interpretation necessarily entails a "I know, I'll tell you" stance, he criticizes a straw man. There are undoubtedly "traditional analysts" who believe that "interpreting things to patients" is an important aspect of the therapeutic process, but who are also very sensitive to the danger of "pulling rank" and of taking an authoritarian "I know, I'll tell you" stance.

In his characterization of the "traditional therapist," Bowlby clearly has in mind the model of the "blank screen" analyst who reads the patient's mind and makes authoritative, "deep" interpretations of the patient's unconscious wishes and fantasies. However, there are many "traditional therapists" who believe that interpretations should be made only when the material interpreted is at the surface of the patient's awareness and who adopt a "you know, you tell me" stance (e.g., Gray, 1990, 1994).

ATTACHMENT THEORY, THERAPEUTIC OUTCOME, AND MEASUREMENT

As noted, Bowlby (1988) states as one of the goals of treatment the restructuring of the patient's representational models of attachment and of current attachment figures (as well as self-representations). One of the primary ways this goal has been concretized in the attachment literature is by identifying the shift from an insecure to a secure attachment pattern as a central outcome goal of treatment, based on the assumption that this shift reflects a change in the patient's underlying representations. In other words, attachment theory enters the picture not in suggesting a particular therapeutic approach, but rather in providing outcome criteria and goals. For example, in the Levy et al. (2006) study discussed in Chapter 4, although attachment status was an outcome criterion, the therapeutic approach employed, transference-focused psychotherapy (TFP), was not derived from attachment theory, but from Kernberg's (1976) version of object relations theory.

The shift from insecure to secure attachment as an outcome of treatment has generally been measured by the AAI. For example, as noted in Chapter 4, in the Levy et al. (2006) study, a substantial number of borderline patients were reported as secure–autonomous on the AAI after one year of TFP treatment. Operationally, this essentially means that the AAI narratives of these patients were more coherent after 1 year of treatment. How does one understand this rather dramatic and surprising finding?

As is the case with any measure, a basic question one needs to consider is the "ecological validity" of the measure employed (see Kazdin, 2006). This question is particularly pertinent in view of the fact that one would not normally expect borderline patients to become securely attached after 1 year of treatment. The critical issue is the relationship between greater coherence on the AAI and secure attachment, as secure attachment is defined by attachment theory. Main et al. (1985) observe that the AAI measures the subject's "state of mind with respect to attachment" (p. 68). However, how AAI categories are related to attachment patterns (and the underlying internal working model), as defined by attachment theory, is an open question. From an attachment theory perspective, the essence of secure attachment is a confident expectation in the availability of the attachment figure as a safe haven in times of distress and as a secure base for exploration. A fundamental validity question for any measure of attachment is its relationship to these essential criteria of secure attachment.

In the Levy et al. (2006) study—and I discuss this study as one arena for examining how to interpret shifts in attachment classifications following treatment—we do not know whether the changes on the AAI indicate that the patients now have a more confident expectation in the availability of their attachment figure as a safe haven and secure base and were, therefore, as Levy et al. put it, better able "to turn to others as a safe haven in times of distress, while when not in distress, utilizing attachment figures as a secure base from which to explore both the physical and the psychological world" (p. 1036) (see also Eagle, 2006). Implicit in Levy et al.'s comments is the idea that the patient's increasing ability to experience the therapist as a safe haven and secure base—as well as a generalization of this experience to attachment figures outside the treatment—would constitute critical attachment outcome criteria for successful treatment.

To sum up, we cannot assume that changes from insecure to secure in AAI classification as an outcome of treatment indicate a shift from insecure to secure attachment. Given the evidence that reflective function and secure base script knowledge account for much of the variance in AAI classifications (see Chapter 4), the shift from insecure to secure on the AAI likely indicates enhanced reflective function and increased secure base script knowledge.

Attachment Pattern and Response to Treatment

There is one area where attachment theory is especially relevant to therapeutic process and outcome. Levy et al. (2011) observe that "attachment organization or style can be a moderator of treatment utilization, outcome, or dropout" (p. 55) and can also be a variable in the interaction between attachment pattern and treatment approach. There is some evidence that the patient's attachment pattern can influence the therapeutic process. For example, Parish and Eagle (2003) found that attachment pattern influenced the intensity of the patient's attachment to the therapist, with, as expected, avoidant patients showing less intense attachment.

As far as therapeutic outcome is concerned, there is some evidence that avoidant–dismissive patients do better in psychotherapy than preoccupied or unresolved patients (Fonagy et al., 1996; McBride, Atkinson, Quilty, & Bagby, 2006). As Slade (2008) notes, these findings may reflect primarily a relationship between degree of psychopathology and therapeutic outcome. That is, compared to avoidant individuals, preoccupied individuals tend to be more disturbed, as evidenced by their overrepresentation in borderline personality disorder (e.g., Agrawal et al., 2004), and by the finding that whereas avoidant attachment is a protective factor, preoccupied attachment in interaction with unresolved-disorganized attachment is a risk factor for suicide (Adam et al., 1996). Also, the finding that preoccupied attachment is associated with greater psychopathology is congruent with the idea that whereas avoidant attachment can be understood in terms of intact defenses, preoccupied attachment can be understood as a partial failure of defense.

The relationship between attachment pattern and therapeutic outcome may also be mediated by the association between attachment pattern and therapeutic alliance. Bachelor, Meunier, Lavardière, and Gamache (2010) found that whereas secure attachment to therapist was significantly associated with a positive alliance, fearful attachment to therapist was predictive of a negative alliance. Furthermore, secure versus fearful attachment was more predictive of therapeutic outcome than personality and symptomatology factors. Finally, it seems to me that although our measures may not be fine enough to capture it, *degree* of avoidance and preoccupation are likely to be important in the relationship between attachment pattern and severity (as well as type) or psychopathology.

The Patient's Attachment Pattern and Therapeutic Approach

The avoidant and the preoccupied patient may present different challenges that may require different therapeutic approaches. As noted, the avoidant patient is more likely to have intact defenses and to minimize the need for help, whereas the preoccupied patient is more overtly anxious and more likely to be more demanding in his or her need for help. Preoccupied attachment was associated with lower therapeutic alliance ratings than either secure or avoidant patients (Mallinckrodt et al., 1995b). Consistent with this finding, Eames and Roth (2000) found that preoccupied patients reported more frequent treatment ruptures, whereas avoidant patients reported fewer ruptures.

There is evidence that the patient's attachment pattern pulls for different responses from the therapist, with the therapist being more likely to employ the more cognitively oriented technique of interpretation with avoidant patients and the more affectively oriented approach of reflection of feelings with preoccupied patients (Hardy et al., 1999; Rubino, Barker, Roth, & Featon, 2000). The relationship of these different approaches to outcome is unknown. Indeed, there is apparently conflicting evidence and views on this issue. Whereas Fonagy et al. (1996) suggested that avoidant patients did better with psychoanalytically oriented psychotherapy, McBride et al. (2006) found that avoidant depressed patients did better with cognitive-behavioral therapy than with interpersonal dynamic theory. Of course, given different diagnostic groups, differences in how treatment approach is implemented, and other differences among these studies, it is difficult to make meaningful comparisons among them. (See Slade, 2008, for an excellent discussion of the relationship between attachment theory and research and adult psychotherapy.)

The Therapist's Attachment Pattern and Therapeutic Process and Outcome

There is also some evidence that the therapist's attachment pattern can influence both the therapeutic process and outcome. For example, Shauenberg et al. (2010) found that although there were no main effects of the therapist's attachment pattern on therapeutic alliance and outcome, higher attachment security was associated with both better alliance and outcome in more disturbed patients. There are a number of studies that investigated the effects of "match" between the patient's and therapist's attachment patterns on therapeutic process and outcome (Dozier, Cue, & Barnett, 1994; Tyrrell, Dozier, & Teague, 1999). In the Tyrrell et al. study, positive outcome was associated with complementarity rather than identity between patient and therapist attachment patterns (e.g., therapist with relatively deactivated pattern paired with patient with relatively hyperactivated attachment pattern vs. both therapist and patient with the same deactivated or hyperactivated attachment pattern). One likely reason that this is so is that there is likely to be less collusion between the patient and therapist (e.g., avoidance of intimacy issues when both patient and therapist are avoidant) when they have different attachment patterns (see also Mohr, Gelso, & Hill, 2005; Rubino et al., 2000; Sauer, Lopez, & Gormley, 2003).

Attachment and Psychotherapy with Couples

I want to briefly discuss attachment-based approaches to work with couples. I focus on the work of Susan Johnson (2008), one of the leading figures in this area. As Johnson notes, difficulties between couples often entail attachment issues and dynamics. She tends to view attachment anxiety and avoidance not so much as trait-like phenomena, but rather as "natural responses" to the lack of a sense of secure connection with one's partner. For Johnson, the experienced failure of one's partner as a reliable safe haven and secure base, particularly during critical times (e.g., parenthood, illness) is the core problem of troubled relationships. Betrayals such as infidelity are seen as essentially attachment injuries.

As for attachment-based interventions, the couple learns that attachment needs are not limited to childhood, but are life-long. Also, the couple therapist needs to help patients to "recognize and 'own' their attachment needs, to guide partners to ask for these needs to be met, in a clear, congruent way that fosters partner responsiveness" (p. 813). This help is partly provided by a focus on emotions such as anger in response to separation, panic in response to rejection, and sadness in response to the experience that one's partner is inaccessible or does not care (p. 814). Johnson's attachment-based emotion-focused therapy (EFT) also includes "a focus and validation of attachment needs and fears, and the promotion of safe emotional engagement, comfort, and support" (p. 821). According to Johnson, "attachment is not used just as an overall perspective on a couple's problems. It also elicits specific interventions." These specific interventions include "empathic reflection of emotional responses and interaction processes, validation and empathic questioning ... used to create a sense of safety and focus the process on attachment needs" (p. 823).

Although it is clear from the above that attachment theory influences the areas on which EFT couple therapy focuses, I have the same problem with viewing EFT interventions as I do with viewing mentalization-based therapy (MBT) or transference-focused psychotherapy (TFP) interventions as specifically derived from attachment theory. Thus, "empathic reflection of emotional responses and interaction processes" or "empathic questioning … used to create a sense of safety" are interventions and stances common to a wide range of therapeutic approaches rather than specifically derived from attachment theory. One way to make the point is to ask whether the rationale for encouraging "empathic reflection of emotional responses and interaction processes" requires attachment theory or whether that rationale would be affected in any way were there no such thing as attachment theory.

Ironically, the near exclusive focus of EFT on *attachment-related content and issues* seems to me to be excessively limiting. There is little doubt that attachment-related issues, such as the degree to which one experiences one's partner as a safe haven and secure base, are core issues in troubled relationships. However, it would seem important to explore further the reason that one may not experience one's partner as a safe haven and secure base. Also, it is likely that attachment issues alone are not always the only or major factor in troubled relationships.

With regard to the first point, one reason that one may not experience one's partner as a safe haven and secure base is that one's partner does not behave in a way that makes it easy to have that experience, that is, is not emotionally available. The issue of object choice becomes especially relevant here. Why does someone choose a mate who cannot readily serve as a safe haven and secure base? Another reason that one may not experience one's partner as a safe haven and secure base is that because he or she is unconsciously equated with one's early rejecting or intrusive or unpredictable attachment figure, one carries over one's early attachment pattern to one's current ongoing relationship. Here, the issue is not so much that one's partner does not serve as a safe haven or secure base, but rather that one assimilates new experiences to old models and schemas. The influence of assimilative processes in how one experiences one's partner is implied in the concept of internal working model and particularly in the idea that it is relatively resistant to change (just as it is implicit in the psychoanalytic concept of transference). One would expect that a couple therapy approach influenced by attachment theory would not only make explicit both partners' implicit internal working models, but would also attempt to clarify the unconscious equation of current partner with early attachment figure (Eagle, 2007).

As for the second point, it seems to me that although attachment issues are extremely important in troubled relationships, other factors may play an important role. For example, Johnson et al. (2006) assume that infidelity is always experienced as an attachment injury, which, indeed, it may be.

However, infidelity is also likely to involve other factors and feelings such as jealousy, humiliation, and perhaps most important, profound betrayal of trust. Also, troubled relationships may involve a variety of other factors, including fear of commitment, anxieties and inhibitions related to Oedipal issues (e.g., experience of sex with partner as forbidden), experience of sex as engulfment, the split between love and desire (Freud, 1912/1957) or equivalently, the split between attachment and sexuality (see Chapter 8)—all of which cannot be subsumed simply under the rubric of attachment issues.

IMPLICATIONS OF ATTACHMENT THEORY FOR CLINICAL INTERVENTIONS WITH INFANT–MOTHER DYADS

I turn now from adult individual and couple psychotherapy to the implications of attachment theory and research for clinical interventions with infant–mother dyads. Although, as Bowlby (1988) notes, attachment is important throughout the lifespan, attachment theory seems especially relevant for understanding and for developing appropriate interventions in regard to the relationship between infant and caregiver. Hence, it should be no surprise that in contrast to adult psychotherapy, the clinical implications of attachment theory and research for interventions with infant–mother dyads are more direct and apparent. And, indeed, a number of infant–mother intervention programs throughout the United States and elsewhere are based on attachment theory whose specific central goal is to enhance the security of the infant's attachment.

If one believes that the child's attachment pattern and underlying internal working model reflect, with reasonable accuracy, interactions with the caregiver (e.g., characterized by sensitive responsiveness vs. rejection); and if one further believes that secure attachment is a protective factor and insecure or disorganized attachment are risk factors, then it seems reasonable that interventions would be geared toward altering these interactions through altering the caregiver's behavior (e.g., from insensitive to sensitive) in the expectation that such changes would increase the likelihood of secure and/or organized attachment in the child. The goals of all infant–mother intervention programs are governed by this rationale.

A good deal of evidence appears to justify this rationale. As we have seen in Chapter 3, secure attachment in infancy is associated with a more favorable developmental trajectory in the areas of cognitive and social functioning and is a protective factor in the development of later psychopathology, whereas insecure attachment and more strongly, disorganized attachment, are associated with a less favorable developmental trajectory and are risk factors for later psychopathology. Hence it would appear to make good sense to set as a central therapeutic goal of intervention programs the enhancement of secure attachment.

Although they may differ somewhat in their foci, virtually all attachment-related infant–mother intervention programs attempt to accomplish this goal through enhancing mother's sensitive responsiveness to her infant. Many intervention programs attempt to do this not through direct manipulation of the mother's behavior, but through enhancing her capacity to reflect on her attitudes toward her child, the way she understands her child's behavior, the links between her attitudes and construals and her own attachment-related early experiences, and the ways in which these attitudes and construals interfere with her ability to accurately read the child's signals and needs and respond appropriately. In short, as Fonagy would put it, these programs are designed to enhance the caregiver's ability to reflect on both her own mental states and those of her child, based on the assumption that such enhancement will increase the likelihood of her sensitive responsiveness and therefore, will strengthen the security of attachment of her child.

Examples of Infant–Mother Intervention Programs

It might be useful at this point to describe briefly a few specific infant–mother intervention programs. (For a more comprehensive and detailed description of infant–mother intervention programs, see Berlin, 2005; Berlin, Zeanah, & Lieberman, 2008.)

CIRCLE OF SECURITY PROGRAM

One of the most carefully thought out of such programs is the "Circle of Security" program developed by Marvin and his colleagues (e.g., 2002) at the University of Virginia. It is a 20-week program that takes place in a group of five or six parents and children from 1 to 4 years of age. The program includes introducing parents to the basic ideas of attachment theory: for example, the needs of the child to explore in an environment in which his or her attachment figure will be available if needed; the need of the child to be comforted, protected, and delighted in; and the importance of repair of disruptions. Parents are helped to understand that, based on their own early experiences, certain needs of their child can activate painful feelings, reactive defense, and miscuing their child about his or her need. The child then adapts to this miscuing by himself or herself miscuing the parent, creating a repetitive vicious circle. The program makes use of video clips of parent–child interactions, interviews, various rating scales, and pre- and postintervention measures. The purpose of the intervention program is to "shift patterns of attachment-caregiving interactions ... to a more appropriate developmental pathway" (p. 107).

In a report of preliminary findings, Hoffman, Marvin, Cooper, and Powell (2006) reported that whereas 80% of the children were classified as insecure in the Strange Situation at preintervention, only 46% were so classified at postintervention. There were also significant decreases in disorganized from pre- to postintervention. The absence of a control group and randomized assignment makes it important to replicate these findings.

CHILD–PARENT PSYCHOTHERAPY OR INFANT–PARENT PSYCHOTHERAPY

This approach is based on Fraiberg's (1980) model, a major premise of which is that difficulties in the infant–mother relationship are largely due to unresolved childhood conflicts and anxieties in relation to the caregiver's own parents. Hence, the major goals of this approach include helping the parent deal with these early anxieties and conflicts and recognize their impact on her relationship with her infant in the context of an empathic and supportive therapist. The interventions are 90-minute home or playroom unstructured sessions once a week for a period of 1 year.

A number of randomized studies that provide evidence for the efficacy of the program have been carried out. In one study, Cicchetti et al. (2006) reported that maltreated children between 12 and 24 months of age, most of whom showed disorganized attachment, were more likely to be securely attached at 26 months of age than control infants after an infant–parent psychotherapy intervention program. However, similar results were found after a home visitation following a psychoeducational parenting intervention which focused on providing educational information "on infant physical and psychological development and parenting, encouraging mothers to seek further education and employment, and enhanced informal social support" (p. 630).

A puzzling finding was that although dramatic postintervention changes in the infants' attachment status occurred, none of the hypothesized variables, such as enhanced maternal sensitivity, changes in maternal representations, parenting attitudes, and social support, was found to be involved in these changes in infant attachment status. Thus, we do not know the processes involved in accounting for the important changes found.

MINDING THE BABY

Minding the Baby is a home visiting program for first-time high-risk mothers, many of whom report a history of trauma. Families are visited weekly by an interdisciplinary team beginning during pregnancy; at 1 year, dyads transition to biweekly visits, which continue to the child's second birthday. The main goals of the intervention are to promote health, attachment, and relationship outcomes through the enhancement of parental reflective functioning (Slade, Sadler, & Mayes, 2005). Preliminary findings show improved health and relationship outcomes, notably higher rates of secure infant attachment and lower rates of disorganized infant attachment, and—in the highest risk mothers—enhanced levels of reflective functioning relative to controls (Slade & Sadler, 2012).

SKILL-BASED TREATMENT

A very brief intervention program has been developed by van den Boom (1994, 1995) for low-income mothers and their 6- to 9-month-old temperamentally irritable infants. It consists of three home visits, each lasting about 2 hours. The focus is on enhancing mothers' responsiveness to their infant's cues. Follow-up assessments were made when the infants were 12, 18, 24, and 42 months of age. At 12 and 18 months, the infants were significantly more likely to be securely attached than control infants. At 18, 24, and 42 months, mothers were significantly more sensitively responsive than control mothers. And at 42 months, there were no significant differences between intervention and control children on an observer-rated Attachment Q-Sort. However, intervention children were significantly more likely to interact harmoniously with an unfamiliar peer.

I want to note here the contribution of psychoanalytic thinking, particularly the work of Fraiberg (1980), to the rationale for many of the intervention programs. This is particularly evident and explicit in the child–parent psychotherapy program of Lieberman and her colleagues, the Circle of Security program of Marvin and his colleagues, and the Minding the Baby program of Slade, Sadler, and colleagues. Thus, one can see that many of the intervention programs designed to enhance security of attachment are based on an amalgam of attachment and psychoanalytic theories.

THE SNUGGLY CARRIER STUDY

Anisfeld, Casper, Nozyce, and Cunningham (1990) reported on the use of a face-to-face Snuggly carrier during the infant's first 4 months of life with high-risk mothers as a means of influencing the infant's security of attachment. Note that unlike virtually all other intervention programs, no attempt was made to enhance the mother's reflective capacity. What is striking is that 84% of Snuggly carrier infants were classified as securely attached in the Strange Situation at 1 year of age, compared to 38% of securely attached infants in the control group (where mothers were given a child plastic seat). This is one of the largest differences found in any intervention program (van IJzendoorn, Juffer, & Duyvesteyn, 1995).

Of course, given how dramatic the effect was, one would want to replicate the study. Nevertheless, one can speculate about the possible factors and processes involved in producing the effect. What is it about carrying the infant in a face-to-face Snuggly carrier a good part of the day for a period of 4 months that may contribute to security of attachment at 1 year of age? For one thing, it provides more kinesthetic and tactile stimulation than would normally be the case. However, very likely other factors are operating. One can hypothesize that prolonged face-to-face contact strengthens the mother's bond to her infant. It is also possible that the Snuggly carrier experience itself enhances the mother's capacity to reflect on her infant's and her own mental states despite the fact that the intervention did not focus on this goal. However, this was not measured in the study. In any replication, one would want to include careful measures of various aspects of the mother's attitudes, representations, and behaviors in relation to her infant. However, at the very least, the Anisfeld et al. (1990) study suggests that there may be more roads to foster infant security of attachment and possibly even many roads to enhance mother's reflective capacity other than attempts to do so directly.

Effectiveness of Preventive and Intervention Programs

How effective are the various preventive and intervention programs that have been implemented? I have addressed this question partially in describing the above programs. However, a more systematic answer is warranted. The general question of effectiveness generates at least three subquestions:

1. How effective are these programs in enhancing the child's attachment security?
2. How effective are these programs in changing the caregiver's representations and behavior, particularly sensitivity?
3. As we have discussed earlier (see Chapter 3), how strong is the relationship between maternal sensitivity and infant or child secure attachment?

In a 1995 review of "attachment-based interventions," van IJzen-doorn et al. found mixed and complex results. Some interventions were associated with greater maternal sensitivity, but there were no measurable effects on infants' security of attachment (e.g., Barnard et al., 1998). In one study, the intervention reduced mother's anxiety, but did not influence infants' attachment status (Barnett, Blignault, Holmes, Payne, & Parker, 1987). Somewhat conversely, Lyons-Ruth et al. (1990) reported that although a weekly home visit intervention with high-risk mothers did not produce changes in maternal sensitivity, it did appear to influence infant security of attachment. In the Anisfeld et al. (1990) intervention described above, a very large effect on infant security of attachment was obtained without observable changes in maternal sensitivity. And finally, van den Boom (1994) reported that an intervention consisting of three or four home visits with mothers of highly irritable infants between 6 and 9 months of age was associated with both greater maternal sensitivity and infant secure attachment at 1 year of age. Van IJzendoorn et al. conclude that enhancing maternal sensitivity does not necessarily change the infant's attachment status—hence, the need to "search for alternative pathways to attachment" (p. 245). One must note, however, the question remains as to how adequately maternal sensitivity has been measured in these studies (see Chapter 3).

Berlin et al., at a later date (2008), also reviewed the research literature on the effectiveness of preventive and intervention programs that attempt to enhance attachment security. Because the intervention programs vary with regard to their focus, age at which intervention is carried out, nature of the sample targeted, duration of the intervention, outcome variables, measurement instruments, and extent of follow-up, there is no simple summary one can cite. For example, some researchers report "more is better" (Egeland, Weinfield, Bosquet, & Cheng, 2000, p. 79); others have concluded that "less is more" (Bakermans-Kranenberg, van IJzendoorn, Pijlman, Mesman, & Juffer, 2003). Both Berlin (2005) and Greenberg (2005) argue that both can be true, depending on the nature of the sample.

Based on a 2005 meta-analysis, Bakermans-Kranenberg et al. conclude that interventions that focus on maternal sensitivity are more effective than interventions that provide support and focus on the parent's working model. However, this conclusion is not congruent with the results of the Snuggly carrier intervention (Anisfeld et al., 1990), which did not involve any direct focus on maternal sensitivity. It is also not congruent with the report by Lieberman, Weston, and Pawl (1991) that a focus on mother's own early experiences (following the Fraiberg, 1980, model) enhanced maternal empathy and involvement and lowered avoidance and anger toward mother—although it did not enhance attachment security as measured by the Attachment Q-sort. The Bakermans-Kranenberg, van IJzendoorn, and Juffer (2005) conclusion is also not compatible with the finding noted above that a child–parent psychotherapy intervention did enhance infant security (Cicchetti et al., 2006)—despite no measurable enhancement of maternal sensitivity (see also Toth et al., 2006)—nor with the Slade & Sadler (2012) finding that focusing on maternal reflective functioning increases rates of infant security.

That there is more than one path to enhanced security of attachment is suggested by van den Boom's (1994, 1995) finding that a relatively short intervention that focused on mothers' sensitive responsiveness was associated not only with increased maternal responsiveness, but also with enhanced infant security of attachment. It should be noted, however, that at 42 months of age, the intervention program children were no more likely to be securely attached (as measured by the Attachment Q-sort) than a control group—although they were significantly more likely to interact harmoniously with an unfamiliar peer.

After reviewing these and other intervention programs, Berlin at el. (2008) conclude that in assessing the effectiveness of intervention programs, one needs to take account of such factors as nature of the families targeted (e.g., high-risk vs. low-risk); infant temperament (e.g., high vs. low irritability); ingredients of the intervention (e.g., feedback; precisely defined versus general goals); and intervener-parent relationship. In general, the critical question—one that is central to evaluating all intervention programs—is what works for whom?

Once again, one has to note the question of the adequacy of measurement of maternal sensitivity (see Chapter 3). Without adequate measures of maternal sensitivity, it is difficult to draw reliable conclusions regarding the impact of enhancing sensitivity on the attachment status of the child. And finally, implicit in De Wolff and van IJzendoorn's (1997) suggestions, is the likely productiveness of investigating the effects of interventions that are intended to enhance maternal behaviors other than sensitivity.

There seems to be a partial disconnect between general findings on the relationship between maternal sensitivity and infant attachment and the emphasis on enhancing sensitivity in intervention programs. If maternal sensitivity accounts for only a modest percentage of the variability in infant attachment status, might it not be more productive to attempt to enhance a range of maternal behaviors that are associated with secure attachment?

An additional factor needs to be taken into account in evaluating the effectiveness of intervention programs, namely, individual differences among infants in their susceptibility to environmental influences (Belsky et al., 2007) (see Chapter 3). Bakermans-Kranenberg et al. (2008) investigated the effectiveness of a video-feedback intervention intended to promote positive parenting and sensitive discipline among 1- to 3-year-olds who were screened for their relatively high levels of externalizing behavior. The authors found that the intervention was effective in decreasing externalizing behavior in children with the dopamine D4 receptor (DRD4) 7-repeat allele, whereas it was not effective in children without the 7-repeat DRD4 allele. They also found that children with the DRD4 7-repeat allele showed lower cortisol levels as a function of the parental video-feedback intervention, whereas this was not the case for the children without the DRD4 7-repeat allele. Such findings suggest that individual differences in susceptibility to environmental influences among infants will moderate the effectiveness of any intervention program. They also suggest that in order to maximize effectiveness, one may need to move from one-size-fits-all intervention programs to programs that take better account of individual differences among infants.

Limitations of Research on Effectiveness of Intervention Programs

A serious limitation of studies assessing the effectiveness of intervention programs is the lack of *follow-up* in two areas. One, we do not know the developmental trajectory of the infants who have become more securely attached through the intervention programs. The implicit assumption seems to be that since, in general, secure attachment has been found to be associated with a more positive developmental trajectory, this will also be true for the infants who have achieved secure attachment in the intervention programs. But we do not know whether this is, in fact, the case. That is, we do not know whether the developmental trajectories of infants who are securely attached without interventions are the same as or similar to those of infants whose secure attachment status is attributable to interventions. We do not even know whether an infant who, through the intervention program, becomes securely attached at the age of 12 or 18 months remains securely attached at later ages of, say, 3 or 4 or 5, or later in life. In only one intervention program described was there a follow-up as late as 42 months.

Related to this question is the question relating to the "lasting power" of interventions that are shown to, in fact, enhance mother's sensitive responsiveness or reflective capacity or other aspects of her behavior. To what extent does mother continue her "gains" beyond the duration of the intervention programs? We know that the requirements of adequate caregiving change along with developmental changes in the child. Is there a carryover from what mother has learned in the intervention program with her 1-year-old to her caregiving when her child is now 3 or 5 or 8 years old? There appears to be an implicit and explicit assumption that, for example, the enhancement of reflective capacity will carry over to later situations. But we do not know if this is the case. Until we know the answers to these questions, it is difficult to fully evaluate the effectiveness of these intervention programs. This is certainly a task for future research.

We know that the path from early attachment status to later development is quite complex and is influenced by a variety of factors, including family environment, socioeconomic conditions, social support, and infant susceptibility to environmental influence. This consideration makes it all the more important to carry out follow-up efforts in intervention research. We also know that a large body of research literature has identified factors other than security of attachment that have a significant influence on development. Future research can be directed toward understanding the interactions between attachment status and other critical factors in influencing development.

CHAPTER 12

Convergence and Integration

As noted in Chapter 1, one of Bowlby's primary motives in developing attachment theory was to align psychoanalytic theory more closely to scientific findings and perspectives from related disciplines, such as ethology and cognitive psychology. In this way, he believed, he could reform psychoanalysis and preserve the insights it offered, while modifying those formulations that he viewed as untenable and based on outmoded perspectives that needed to be replaced.

Although the crucible for the origins of attachment theory was psychoanalysis, the fact is that attachment research and theory have developed quite independently of psychoanalysis. According to Fonagy (2001), as I have stated, there is "bad blood" between them. In rather stark contrast to the embeddedness of psychoanalysis in clinical work, attachment theory has been closely linked to systematic empirical research, which is generally published not in psychoanalytic but in psychology journals and is carried out by researchers, many of whom have no particular interest in psychoanalysis. In short, attachment theory and research have developed quite independently of psychoanalysis. Nevertheless, as we will see, there are important areas of possible mutual contributions as well as potential convergence and integration between these two perspectives.

My purpose in this final chapter is to identify and discuss these mutual contributions and to point to convergences and possibilities of greater integration between these two perspectives. Fonagy has provided an excellent chapter entitled "What Do Psychoanalytic Theories and Attachment Theory Have in Common?" in his 2001 book *Attachment and Psychoanalysis*. Fonagy focuses on the common emphasis on the importance of early caregiving; the role of mentalization; the conception of representations of self and other as determinants of interpersonal behavior; the relationship context of cognitive development; and the fundamental motivations for forming relationships. I will not duplicate his efforts. Rather, I limit my discussion to selected points of convergence between attachment and psychoanalytic theories that supplement Fonagy's chapter. Even when I do discuss the same topics covered by Fonagy, I do so from a somewhat different perspective. The topics I discuss in this chapter are (1) the basis for infant–mother attachment; (2) the importance of mentalization and reflective function in classical and contemporary psychoanalytic theories; (3) the role of adequate caregiving in optimal development; (4) the role of fantasy and actual events in influencing representations and development; (5) restrictions on experience; (6) persistence of early modes of relating; (7) ego functions and attachment; and (8) interpersonalizing of defense.

THE BASIS FOR INFANT–MOTHER ATTACHMENT

I have already noted in previous chapters various points of convergence between attachment theory and psychoanalysis. They include, for example, an emphasis on early experiences in influencing personality development and the role of the therapist as a base from which the patient can engage in self-exploration.

Also, as noted in Chapter 1, Bowlby (1958) identified early psychoanalytic precursors to attachment theory. They include Ferenczi's (1933) concept of "passive object love"; Balint's (1937) concept of "primary object love," which according to him is not linked to any of the erotogenic zones "but is something, on its own" (p. 15); Hermann's (1933, 1936) positing of an instinct to cling; and Suttie's (1935/1988) identification of "instincts adapted to infancy," the predominant component of which is "a simple attachment to mother" (p. 15).

Bowlby also notes that when Burlingham and Freud (1944) actually observed children, their descriptions are quite different from Anna Freud's theoretical formulations, which stress hunger reduction and the pleasures associated with infantile sexuality as the basis for attachment. For example, based on the observations of children in the Hampstead Nurseries, they write that "children will cling even to mothers who are continually cross and sometimes cruel to them. The attachment of the small child to his mother seems to a large degree independent of her personal qualities" (p. 47). In that same paper, they describe the child's need "for early attachment as an important instinctual need" (p. 22).

As is the case with Burlingham and Freud, when Klein actually observes infants, her descriptions are quite different from her theoretical formulations. Bowlby cites the following passage from Klein's writings:

> Some children who, although good feeders, are not markedly greedy, show unmistakable signs of love and of a developing interest in the mother at very early stages—an attitude which contains some essential elements of an object-relation. I have seen babies as young as three weeks interrupt their sucking for a short time to play with the mother's breast or to look towards her face. I have also observed that young infants—even as early as in the second month—would in wakeful periods after the feeding lie on the mother's lap, look up at her, listen to her voice and respond to it by their facial expression; it was like a loving conversation between mother and baby. Such behavior implies that gratification is as much related to the object, which gives the food as to the food itself. (Klein et al., 1952, p. 239)

Bowlby cites Ribble's (1943) conclusion that there is an "innate need for contact with the mother" (Bowlby, 1958, p. 373), but notes that she links this need to "satisfactory functioning of physiological processes" (p. 373) rather than "a social bond developing in its own right" (p. 373). Here, it seems to me, Bowlby, does not fully appreciate Ribble's prescience in anticipating the idea that the mother's role in regulating the infant's physiological (and correspondingly affective) processes may constitute a basis for later psychological attachment to mother—a formulation more fully developed in the work of Hofer and his colleagues (see Chapter 3).

Bowlby also notes Freud's flirtations—and they are only flirtations that are not developed further—with the idea that the infant's attachment to mother may be independent of both hunger reduction and pleasures from erogenous zones. As we have seen in Chapter 8, Freud (1912/1957) refers to the "affectionate current" that is directed to "members of the family and those who look after the child" and "corresponds to the child's primary object choice" (pp. 180–181).

Freud suggests that the "affectionate current, which is 'older' and predates the 'sensual' current, is the basis for the infant's primary object choice." As I have noted elsewhere, "Freud, in effect, is proposing that the infant's attachment to the caregiver is based on a system that predates and that, therefore, is initially independent of infantile sexuality" (Eagle, 2007, pp. 46–47). Freud does not further develop the implications of this proposal. Had he done so, he might have abandoned his secondary drive theory and more fully anticipated important aspects of attachment theory.

THE IMPORTANCE OF MENTALIZATION AND REFLECTIVE FUNCTIONING CAPACITY IN ATTACHMENT THEORY AND CLASSIC PSYCHOANALYTIC THEORY

Distinction between Mentalization and Reflective Function

In this section I discuss the common emphasis on the importance of mentalization and reflective capacity in optimal functioning in both classical psychoanalytic theory and attachment theory. Before doing so, however, I want to make what I believe is an important distinction between mentalization and reflective function. According to Jurist et al. (2008), "the construct of reflective functioning ... is essentially an operationalization of mentalization" (p. 2). But, it seems that this cannot be right for a number of reasons. Mentalization refers to the capacity to take an "intentional stance" (Dennett, 1987) toward oneself and others, that is, to view behavior in terms of mental states (i.e., aims, intentions, desires, etc.) that the behaviors convey. As Bateman and Fonagy (2006) put it, "mentalizing simply implies a focus on mental states in oneself or in others, particularly in explanations of behavior" (p. 1). As Bateman and Fonagy also note, "mentalization is procedural, mostly non-conscious" (p. 3). Further, Gergely and Unoka (2008) argue that research suggests that mentalization begins as early as 1 year of age.

One would surely not want to say that *reflecting* on one's own and others' mental states is mostly nonconscious or that it begins at 1 year of age. In short, one can mentalize in the sense of (often automatically) taking an intentional stance toward oneself and others without necessarily reflecting on what one has mentalized. As we see later in the chapter, strong unregulated affects are often triggered by automatic attribution of hostile and rejecting intentions to others, which then justifies one's own hostile intentions (see Dodge et al., 1995). In these instances, an intentional stance *is* taken by the individual. That is, the other's behavior is, indeed, explained by reference to his or her intentions and aims. Failure to take an intentional stance is not the problem. The problem is (1) that the attribution of intentions to the other is fixed and rigid and not infrequently, the product of projection and (2) that the individual is not able to *reflect* on his or her attributions, that is, on what he or she has mentalized. Not uncommonly, a vicious circle develops characterized by (1) the triggering of strong negative affects resulting from particular attributions to the other, (2) the failure to reflect on one's attributions due, in part, to the experience of intense negative affect, and (3) attributions that remain unquestioned and continue to "justify" intense negative affect.

Mentalization, Attachment Theory, and Psychoanalysis

Whether or not mentalization-based therapy is based on attachment theory (see Chapter 10), there is nevertheless convergence between classical psychoanalytic theory and attachment theory on the enhancement of reflective functioning as a central therapeutic goal. As Allen, Fonagy, and Bateman (2008) observe, although Freud did not use the term "mentalizing," he essentially originated the concept in his early writings. For example, in his conception of the somatic symptoms of hysteria, he placed great stress on the importance of transforming the somatic into thought—which can be seen as an early precursor of the goal of making the unconscious conscious (see Bucci, 1997, for a contemporary version of the transformation of the subsymbolic into the symbolic as the core psychoanalytic goal). Mentalization is also implicit in Freud's discussion of the origin of thinking and in the importance of inserting thought between impulses and action. This is yet another precursor of the goal of making the unconscious conscious understood as the transformation of what is not thought into what is thought.

In the clinical psychoanalytic context, the role of reflective function is perhaps most clearly expressed in the primacy of strengthening the observing function of the ego as a central treatment goal (Sterba, 1934). This is an especially important idea insofar as it emphasizes the enhancement of an ego function rather than the bringing of specific repressed memories, wishes, and fantasies into consciousness. This change in emphasis from uncovering repressed mental contents to enhancing the observing function of the ego is succinctly captured in the shift from making the unconscious conscious to "where id was, there shall ego be" (Freud, 1933, p. 80) as a central goal of psychoanalytic treatment. The emphasis is now not only or perhaps not primarily on bringing material to consciousness, but also on reflecting on what is now in conscious awareness. Insofar as one can understand reflective capacity as an ego function, the goal of strengthening ego functions includes the enhancement of mentalization and reflective capacity. Recent work on mentalization at least partly inspired by attachment theory expands the psychoanalytic goal of strengthening the observing function of the ego by including in that function the capacity to reflect on the mental states of others.

The Importance of Reflective Function in Later Psychoanalytic Theories

The emphasis on enhancing reflective function—even if that term may not be employed—comes to the fore and becomes increasingly explicit in the work of those contemporary analysts who focus on analysis of defense. In the view of contemporary ego psychologists such as Gray (1994), Sugarman (2006), and Busch (2009), the main function of interpretation is not to uncover repressed wishes and fantasies, but to enhance the patient's curiosity about and capacity for understanding how his or her mind works. In effect, Gray and his colleagues are describing mentalization and reflective function.

An assumption shared by both attachment theory and psychoanalysis is that enhancement of the capacity for reflection serves as an affect regulator and as a barrier against the "thoughtless" automatic repetition of maladaptive patterns. Many patients, particularly those suffering from borderline and narcissistic disorders, tend to construe and experience the behavior of others as rejecting, humiliating, and so on (see Gunderson & Lyons-Ruth, 2008, for evidence that borderline patients are rejection sensitive). Their reactions to such experiences often trigger uncontrollable negative affects and wreak havoc in their relationships.

This phenomenon is nicely illustrated in a clinical example provided by Gabbard and Horowitz (2009). The patient reports an incident in which she experienced a sales clerk's refusal to accept her credit card as an affront and reacted by creating a scene in the store. In response to her therapist's question as to whether the sales clerk's refusal to accept her credit card was store policy, the patient reacts with rage, accusing her therapist of taking the sales clerk's side. In the throes of her emotional reaction, she does not seem capable of reflecting on her construal of the sales clerk's intentions.

In my own clinical work I have been struck with the frequency with which these unquestioned attributions to others of intentions to humiliate are made, their role in triggering a spiral of destructive negative affects and behaviors, and the affect-regulating efficacy of reflecting on these attributions. As an example of these phenomena, a patient reported her father's response to her phone call to pick her up at the train station with the suggestion that she take a taxi (because he was having his dinner) as an egregious example of his rejection of her. In the past, this sort of experience would lead to the following sequence: rage, accompanied by such thoughts as "I never want to see him again. I don't need him. I don't need anybody"; inability to sustain these "resolutions"; feeling "weak" and dependent; depression; suicidal thoughts. During this session (after a good deal of previous work), she was able to reflect on both her own feelings of rejection and her own wishes in relation to her father as well as on her father's perspective (i.e., his wish to eat his dinner rather than his intention to reject her or his not caring about her). This newfound capacity for mentalization and reflection—which my patient described as her new "tool"—served to prevent the destructive sequence I have described above.

Both Gabbard and Horowitz's patient and my patient, in her initial construal of her father's behavior, *are* mentalizing in the sense that they are attributing aims and intentions to the other—intentions to reject and humiliate, for example. However, they experience their own reactions as well as their attributions to the other as absolute and unquestioned, and not subject to evaluation and reflection. Hence, their failure lies not in an incapacity to mentalize, but in a relative incapacity to reflect on what they mentalize.

One can see in these examples another phenomenon highlighted by Fonagy and his colleagues, namely, either the interference with mentalization or the increased rigidity of reflective function when strong affect is aroused. In the case of my patient, the intense affect is clearly related to the activation of her attachment system, that is, wanting her father to be there as a safe haven.

One can also observe failures of reflective function when an individual engages in projection. That is, one projects, say, a hostile wish on to another, then attributes hostility to the other, and then experiences the other as hostile. The one doing the projecting is engaging in mentalization, that is, is taking an "intentional stance"; he or she is attributing certain intentions and aims to the other. However, he or she has not been capable of reflecting on either his or her own or the other's mental states. The projector does not reflect on the possibility that he or she may be angry and that his or her attribution of hostility to the other may be mistaken (or perhaps induced by his or her own behavior).

As we have seen, the caregiver's failure to reflect on either her own or her infant's mental states is hypothesized to contribute to the infant's insecure attachment. Another factor is the tendency of the caregiver to project conflict-laden thoughts, feelings, and motives on to her infant. Recall Lieberman's (1999) description of an interaction in which mother, who is having her lunch, keeps her hungry crying infant, whom she describes as "greedy," waiting until she finishes her own lunch. It is apparent from the material that mother unconsciously views her own neediness as greed and projects these feelings on to her infant. Here, once again, the problem lies not in incapacity to mentalize or take an "intentional stance." Indeed, mother overattributes intentions and feelings to her infant. The problem is that mother is not aware that the intentions and feelings attributed to her infant have little to do with what the infant is intending and feeling. Rather, they are projections of mother's intentions and feelings—a quintessential example of bringing "ghosts into the nursery" (Fraiberg, Adelson, & Shapiro, 1975). Thus, mother's behavior can be understood as a form of mentalization—or perhaps one should say pseudomentalization—in which, although an intentional stance is taken, the intentions attributed to the other are projections of one's own.

One sees a similar pattern in child abuse in which the caregiver attributes to the infant motives and intentions that are "complementary" to and serve to justify the caregiver's negative reactions to the infant. For example, if the caregiver is enraged by the infant's incessant crying, it follows that the infant is *intending* to harass and enrage her by continuing to cry. Again, this is not a matter of failure to take an intentional stance, but rather a matter of overattributing intentions that serve to justify one's own mental state.

THE ROLE OF ADEQUATE CAREGIVING IN OPTIMAL DEVELOPMENT

Convergence between Attachment Theory and Winnicott's Formulations

As Fonagy (2001) notes, a "radical claim" made by Winnicott (1965) is that the development of the child's ego functions is influenced by the caregiver's responses to the child, a claim that accords with the evidence that the caregiver's sensitive responsiveness influences the development of the child's cognitive functioning. Although few would be surprised by this relationship today, Fonagy quite rightly refers to Winnicott's claim as a "radical" new one.

As discussed in Chapter 3, according to psychoanalytic ego psychology, cognitive functions could develop autonomously of drive gratification in an "average expectable environment" (Hartmann, 1958). This acknowledgment of the autonomy of ego functions was heralded as an advance in psychoanalytic theorizing that reflected what we had learned about autonomous and genetically programmed maturational processes. Although psychoanalytic theorists, such as Spitz, for example, were certainly aware of the dire effects of environments outside the average expectable range—maternal deprivation is an obvious example—little attention was paid to the possibility that subtle variations *within* an "average expectable environment" may produce individual differences in cognitive (and social) functioning. In other words, drawing upon attachment theory and employing the language of psychoanalytic theory, one can say that although ego functioning may develop autonomously in relation to drive gratification, it is nevertheless influenced by variations in object relations within the boundaries of an "average expectable range."

Points of Convergence between Kohut's Self Psychology and Attachment Theory

The importance of the caregiver's sensitive responsiveness for the development of secure attachment in attachment theory and Kohut's (1984) emphasis on parental empathic understanding in the development of a cohesive self represent a clear case of a general convergence. However, whether there is a more fine-grained convergence between the two perspectives can only be determined by comparing the specific behavioral and personality characteristics that each perspective emphasizes. Attachment theory identifies insecure attachment as a consequence of lack of parental responsiveness, whereas self psychology focuses on the lack of self-cohesiveness as a consequence of lack of parental empathic mirroring and understanding. Is there a relationship between insecure attachment and lack of self-cohesiveness? How would the latter be assessed? Would operationalizing empathic mirroring and sensitive responsiveness point to the same or different aspects of parental behavior?

As we have seen in previous chapters, attachment research has shown that insecure and particularly disorganized attachment are predictive of a range of certain maladaptive cognitive and social behaviors as well as increased risk for certain forms of psychopathology. According to self-psychology theory, failure to develop a cohesive self is also correlated with certain behaviors (e.g., grandiosity) as well as increased proneness to certain forms of psychopathology (e.g., narcissistic personality disorder). What is the relationship between these two sets of correlates and predictions? Until these questions are empirically investigated, we do not know the specific degree of convergence between self psychology and attachment theory.

THE ROLE OF FANTASY AND ACTUAL EVENTS IN INFLUENCING REPRESENTATIONS AND DEVELOPMENT

The longstanding debate between attachment theory and psychoanalysis on the role of fantasy versus actual events in shaping development merits further discussion and unpacking. I will try to show that there are certain points of convergence (as well as divergence) between these two perspectives. As noted in a previous chapter, I do not think it is true that Kleinian and Freudian theory totally ignore the role of actual events or that attachment theory totally overlooks the role of fantasy. The differences between them are more subtle than that.

A careful reading of Bowlby's objections to Kleinian theory suggests that they can be broken down into a number of explicit and implicit components which, though related to each other, are nevertheless separable. One component is the criticism that Kleinian theory ignores the role of actual events in the development of the infant and child. A second component is the criticism that Kleinian theory places an excessive emphasis on the role of fantasy in understanding the infant's and child's development and psychological life. A third more implicit component is the rejection of the Kleinian assumption that the infant's and child's fantasies are generated, not by actual events, but by *endogenous* drives, particularly the death instinct. A fourth, also implicit, component is the skepticism directed toward the kind of florid and complex fantasies attributed to infants by Klein and Kleinian theorists. I think one can add a fifth component, which consists in Bowlby's claim that from the start that infant is capable of reality testing rather than having to rely on a complex set of projective and introjective processes in order to "construct" an external world. These latter components may not have been all explicitly stated by Bowlby. However, I believe that they are at least implicit aspects of Bowlby's general attitude and skepticism toward Kleinian theory.

Not all the above criticisms are equally justifiable. The passage cited from Rivière in Chapter 1, and Bowlby's response to it ("role of environment = 0") notwithstanding, as we have seen in a previous chapter, Kleinian theory does not discount the role of actual events in the development of the child. Although the emphasis on endogenous instincts remains, an assumption of Kleinian theory is that one needs good object experiences in order to modulate hate and destructiveness emanating from the death instinct and to strengthen object love and the life instinct. For example, as Segal (1964) writes, "when there is a predominance of good experience over bad experience, the ego acquires a belief in the prevalence of the ideal object over the persecutory objects, and also the predominance of its own life instinct over its own death instinct" (p. 24). Although this may not be the role that Bowlby would give to actual experience, it certainly does not entail an utter neglect of actual events.

In its reaction against Kleinian theory, attachment theory appears to leave little room for the role of fantasy of any kind as well as the idiosyncratic ways in which the child may experience actual events—what in the psychoanalytic context is referred to as "psychic reality." By calling attention to fantasy and the idiosyncratic ways in which the child experiences actual events, I do not have in mind the florid fantasies of the devouring breast or urethral attacks attributed to the infant by Klein. There is not an iota of evidence for the existence of such fantasies (how would one even obtain such evidence?); and everything that we know about the infant's capacities—as impressive as they are—strongly suggests that they are not capable of such cognitive activities. What I have in mind is the role of such factors as immature cognition and temperament in influencing how actual events are experienced by the infant and child. It is likely, for example, that infants with different thresholds for frustration will encode the same objective event (e.g., number of minutes waiting to be fed) differently (Eagle, 1995). We also know that young children often understand events in idiosyncratic ways. For example, a young child may experience a caregiver's depression as rejection and/or as caused by his or her demands. Or he or she may experience parental divorce as his or her fault. Also, as Fairbairn (1952) observes, the young child may experience himself or herself as "bad" in order to maintain a representation of the caregiver as "good" and thus keep some semblance of hope alive.

Bowlby himself, as well as attachment theorists and researchers, appear to recognize and acknowledge that representation of early experiences are not simply accurate records of actual events. Bowlby (1973) notes, for example, the existence of incompatible representational models, only one of which—the unconscious one—reflects what the child actually experienced. The other conscious representational model, Bowlby tells us, reflects parental communications that may or may not be congruent with the child's experiences. For example, the child may have felt rejected by his or her caregiver, while at the same time being told by the caregiver what a loving mother she is.[1] Thus, the individual's conscious working model may include the fantasy of a perfectly loving mother. One sees this phenomenon in the idealization of the parental figure seen in AAI narratives (unaccompanied by specific episodic instantiations) as well as the parental idealization often observed in mistreated and abused children.

Thus, even from the perspective of attachment theory, it is not the case that representations reflect, simply and directly, early actual events or early actual experiences. The conscious representational model based on parental communications to which Bowlby refers hardly reflects actual events with "tolerable accuracy." Rather, it is the "distorted" and fantasy-influenced product of the defense against the anxiety generated by parental

---

[1]Bowlby (1973) states that "the hypothesis of multiple models, one of which is highly influential but relatively or completely unconscious, is no more than a version, in different terms, of Freud's hypothesis of a dynamic unconscious" (p. 205).

prohibitions and threats to the relationship with the attachment figure. For example, the threats may take the form of implicitly demanding "that the child accept the parental version by threatening to abandon or eject him, or else to become ill or commit suicide" (Bowlby, 1973, p. 318). In effect, Bowlby is acknowledging the role of defense and fantasy in influencing the child's representational model. What he insists on—in my view, justifiably—is that the child's defenses and fantasies are generated not solely or mainly by endogenous drives, but by actual experiences with caregivers. One can capture the essential difference here between Kleinian theory and attachment theory by saying that whereas in the former, reality is constructed (through projection and introjection processes) out of fantasy (that is, linked to endogenous instincts and drives), from an attachment theory perspective, fantasy develops out of the elaborations of experience of actual events in reality. This perspective is also shared by a number of contemporary psychoanalytic theories.[2]

Consider as a concrete example the concept of castration anxiety. According to the classical psychoanalytic view, during the Oedipal phase of psychosexual development, the boy experiences incestuous wishes toward mother and hostile or death wishes toward father. These wishes are endogenously generated in the course of psychosexual development. Castration anxiety is experienced as a feared retribution for harboring these wishes. According to the traditional view, although parental threats may occur, castration anxiety need not entail actual specific parental threats of castration. Rather, it may be based mainly on the child's fantasy of the kind of punishment that would fit the crime.

Contrast this view with Weiss and Sampson's (1986) understanding of this phenomenon. First, they refer to castration anxiety as a general metaphor for the child's fear of bodily harm associated with "dangerous" and forbidden strivings. Most important, these strivings are not necessarily inherently dangerous but have been rendered so through parental communications. Thus, based on these communications, a child may experience normal ambitions and strivings for independence and separation as entailing harm to parents.

On Weiss and Sampson's view, this is not because the child necessarily

---

[2]There is somewhat of a contradiction in Kleinian theory regarding the role of external reality, including actual events, in external reality, in psychological functioning. On the one hand, as noted above, there is the recognition that actual events, such as good object experiences, can modulate and temper the impact of the death instinct. However, if reality is constructed out of and is the product of projective and introjective processes, then there are no actual events that are even relatively independent of the projection and introjection of fantasies linked to life and death instincts and could therefore contribute to the construction of external reality.

has fundamental and inherent antisocial wishes to harm the parent, but because the parent has communicated the message to the effect that "if you separate and lead an independent life, you will be destroying me," or, to take another example, "if you succeed in your ambitions and outdo me, you will cause me great harm." In other words, the child's unconscious representations and beliefs now include *symbolic equivalences* between certain strivings and harming parents (Eagle, 1987).

Weiss (1982) describes a patient whose father was crippled in an automobile accident when the patient was 5 years old and when he was struggling to be independent. There was evidence that the young boy developed the belief that his attempt to become independent somehow caused his father's disability, and he continued to associate his striving for independence with harm to his father. One can speculate that the young boy's construal of the meaning of his father's accident was, at least in large part, a product not only of immature cognition and the time in his life at which the accident occurred (i.e., when he was striving for independence), but also of the pre-accident parental communication conveying the message that striving for independence was somehow harmful to father.

One can think of these "symbolic equivalences" as fantasies based on actual events. For example, following, say, father's depression or competitiveness or anger following a child's expressions of ambition or outstanding achievement, he or she may come to feel that there is something inherently dangerous or bad or destructive about being ambitious and excelling. Although the father's depression or competitiveness following the child's achievements are actual events, the child may elaborate in fantasy the dangerousness or "badness" of his or her ambitions and strivings.

Consider as another example a child's "average expectable" neediness being met with a response of irritability and tiredness from a depressed parent. The child may develop a symbolic equivalence between expression of his or her normal needs and harming and displeasing parent in some way. Furthermore, the degree of harm to parent may be greatly elaborated in fantasy such that any feeling or expression of need is unconsciously experienced as destroying the other (see Fairbairn, 1952).

In summary, an attachment theory perspective is virtually identical with the view of those contemporary psychoanalytic theorists who reject Freud's positing of universal endogenous antisocial fantasies and wishes that need to be tamed. Instead, they emphasize the role of parental threats and prohibitions in relation to the child's pursuit of basic needs and normal strivings, which are then experienced as "dangerous," conflictual, anxiety-laden, and not to be consciously pursued or experienced. However, what is underemphasized in an attachment theory perspective is the degree to which fantasy elaborations of actual events may contribute to anxiety-laden representations.

It seems to me that the differences between the Kleinian and Freudian theory and attachment theory—as well as the differences between Freudian and Kleinian theory and some contemporary psychoanalytic theories—are not simply a matter of fantasy versus actual events. Rather, the differences have mainly to do with the origins, nature, and role of fantasy in the life of the child. To some extent, these differences reflect fundamentally different conceptions of human nature.

RESTRICTIONS ON EXPERIENCE:
WHAT IS THE CHILD NOT ALLOWED TO THINK AND FEEL?

A central point made by Bowlby is that the anxiety generated by fear of loss, rejection, and threats to the attachment bond influence what one is "allowed" to consciously think and feel . Whatever other differences there are between them, in an important sense, Bowlby's emphasis on parental communications in influencing what the child can and cannot experience is entirely compatible with Freud's discussion of the role of the "danger situations" (e.g., loss of the object; loss of the object's love) in keeping certain thoughts and feelings from being consciously experienced. Where they differ is their sharply different ideas on (1) what thoughts and feelings parents are telling the child he or she is not allowed to consciously experience and (2) the origin and nature of these thoughts and feelings. For Freud, parental prohibitions and threats are directed toward the child's endogenously generated sexual and aggressive thoughts and feelings. The classic example is, of course, the incestuous and hostile wishes that make up the Oedipus complex. Further, according to Freudian theory, in prohibiting these thoughts and feelings and withdrawing love when they are expressed, parents are carrying out a necessary *socializing* function as societal surrogates.

In contrast, for Bowlby, parental prohibitions, threats, and related communications are directed, not toward endogenously generated sexual and aggressive wishes, but toward such aspects of the child's life as wanting to be fed on time (see Lieberman, 1999), wanting to be soothed and comforted, wanting to be accepted and loved, and wanting to have the attachment figure available as a secure base for exploration. In addition, as we have seen, according to Bowlby, parental prohibitions and communications are also directed toward protecting their image as loving parents. To be noted here is that in stark contrast to the Freudian view, little in attachment theory speaks to the socializing function of parental prohibitions and threats. Attachment theory does not appear to posit inherently unruly asocial or antisocial urges and impulses that require parental threats and prohibitions to be tamed and socialized.

PERSISTENCE OF EARLY MODES OF RELATING

Common to attachment theory and psychoanalysis is the assumption that a central feature of psychopathology is the persistence of early modes of relating which, whatever adaptive purposes they may have served in childhood, have become maladaptive. However, attachment theory and psychoanalysis account for the persistence of early modes of relating in different ways. According to attachment theory, these patterns were originally motivated by attempts to have one's attachment needs met in whatever way possible and to avoid the pain of rejection. However, over time they have become habitual and persist into adulthood.

According to Fairbairn (1952), the persistence of early modes of relating is motivated by the individual's "devotion" and "obstinate attachment" to early objects (a phenomenon one often sees in clinical work). From Fairbairn's perspective, the persistence of early modes of relating, which would presumably also include early attachment patterns, is a way of maintaining a kind of loyalty and connection to early objects. Such "devotion" and "obstinate attachment," Fairbairn tells us, provides a sense of inner cognitive and affective connection that is necessary for ego functioning. As Jones (1952) writes in the preface to Fairbairn's book:

> If it were possible to condense Dr. Fairbairn's new ideas into one sentence, it might run somewhat as follows: Instead of starting, as Freud did, from stimulation of the nervous system proceeding from excitation of various erotogenous zones and internal tension arising from gonadic activity, Dr. Fairbairn starts at the centre of the personality, the ego, and depicts its strivings and difficulties in its endeavor to reach an object where it may find support. (p. v)

According to Fairbairn, the direst psychological state that an individual can face is to experience an empty inner world devoid of inner connections to objects. Therefore, we cling to any objects, including "bad" objects. Note that for Fairbairn the function of the object and object relations goes beyond the provision of soothing and comforting (the safe haven function) or of a secure base for exploration. A challenge for future work is the integration of this fundamental function of the object identified by

Fairbairn into an attachment theory conceptualization of the functions of the attachment figure.

Kohut's (1984) identification of the role of the object—or as he puts it, the selfobject—in maintaining self-cohesiveness and self-esteem also speaks to an important function of the attachment figure that goes beyond issues of "felt security" and the provision of a safe haven and secure base. Again, one can ask whether this aspect of the function of the attachment figure can be integrated into attachment theory and research.

There is little doubt that one confronts in clinical work the kinds of phenomena identified in Fairbairn's and Kohut's formulations. That is, one sees patients who are intensely attached to an attachment figure who does not seem to be available as either a safe haven or secure base, but is nevertheless experienced, as one of my patients put it, as a "lifeline," as vital to self-integrity and intactness. This kind of profound and intense attachment, which seems related to and yet appears to go beyond the safe haven and secure base functions of the attachment figure identified by attachment theory, needs to be more fully understood and integrated into attachment theory and research.

On a less intense and dramatic level, it is not uncommon in clinical work to encounter patients whose clinging to their attachment figure, despite much conflict and distress, seems to be maintained by the fantasy that someday and somehow they will get what they need from him or her—that is, as one of my patients ironically put it, that they will "live happily ever after." What is striking about this wan and poignant hope is its utter contrast with the stark reality of the actual relationship. Striking—and clinically most compelling—is the persistence of this fantasy, the intense longing accompanying it, and the profound feeling expressed by the patient in one way or another—that life would indeed be bleak and virtually not worth living were this fantasy to be relinquished. What makes this clinical pattern especially relevant to attachment theory is that it appears to be present virtually exclusively in relation to the patient's attachment figure.

Fairbairn (1952) refers to the alluring or exciting as well as rejecting aspects of the attachment figure (of course, he does not use the term "attachment figure"). According to Fairbairn, from an intrapsychic perspective, what truly constitutes a "bad" object is not simply rejection, but the combination of promise or allure and rejection. This sets up an inner state in which one cannot relinquish the fantasy that the object (i.e., attachment figure) will someday fulfill that promise. Furthermore, the individual's affective life is organized around this fantasy, the relinquishment of which is, as noted, often experienced as an unbearable loss. Hence, the individual clings to the object despite much suffering. Mitchell (1988) goes further in suggesting that it is the very suffering that contributes to the tenacity of the attachment bond because it serves to preserve the continuity, connections, familiarity of one's personal, "interactional world" (p. 33).

EGO FUNCTIONS AND ATTACHMENT

Freud linked the development of cognition and reality testing to drive gratification, specifically, to the failure of wishful hallucination to gratify the hunger drive. As a "corrective" to this formulation, psychoanalytic ego psychologists reorganized autonomous ego functions such as competence and mastery (Hendricks, 1943; White, 1959, 1960). Most important, Hartmann (1958) proposed that in an "average expectable environment," ego functions would develop as part of a normal maturational process.

What ego psychology did not do was (1) link the development of ego functions to the availability of the attachment figures and (2) link individual differences in ego functions to variations in the degree and nature of the attachment figure's availability. It was left to attachment theory to recognize that successful exploration of the world—a critical aspect of ego functioning and reality-testing—requires the availability of the attachment figure and the exercise of his or her secure base function. This function of the attachment figure finds no clearly articulated counterpart in classical theory or, as I understand them, in ego psychology, self psychology, or relational psychoanalysis. This constitutes an important contribution of attachment theory and research to an understanding of the development of ego functions.

As noted previously, Hartmann's formulation of ego autonomy in an "average expectable environment" did not seem to include the recognition that variations in caregiving behavior within an "average expectable environment" can have an impact on the development of ego functions and on the child's capacity for relatively comfortable exploration of the world. Thus, whereas ego functions could be autonomous in the sense of relative independence from drive, attachment research has shown that they are not fully autonomous in the sense of relative independence from the vicissitudes of infant–mother interaction.

As discussed earlier, the consequences of extreme maternal deprivation of which Spitz and other ego psychologists were aware were outside the range of an "average expectable environment." What they were not apparently aware of were the more subtle effects on ego functioning of variations and patterns of infant–caregiver interactions that lay *within* the "average expectable environment." These variations and patterns of caregiving do not determine whether ego functions will develop. That is a matter of normal maturational processes (in that sense they are autonomous). However, as a great deal of attachment research has shown, they do influence the way that ego functions such as cognitive and social abilities and defensive patterns develop. Here is obviously another area where attachment theory and research findings have important implications for psychoanalytic theory, in particular, for a theory of the nature and development of ego functions.

INTERPERSONALIZING OF DEFENSE

Although, according to a classic psychoanalytic view, defense originates in interactional experiences (e.g., the child's response to the "danger situations"), once they are established, they are essentially intrapsychic processes. For example, repression operates intrapsychically to keep certain thoughts and feelings from being consciously experienced. And, in adapting the concept of repression to attachment theory, Bowlby (1988) also describes avoidant attachment pattern as an intrapsychic process entailing "defensive exclusion" of attachment-related thoughts and feelings.

However, attachment patterns as defenses also include interpersonal communications and behaviors that have interpersonal consequences. For example, an avoidant attachment pattern entails certain *behaviors*, such as avoidance of intimacy, behaviors that trigger prophecy-fulfilling complementary responses in others, such as withdrawal and rejection. The interpersonal nature and consequences of the enmeshed/preoccupied attachment pattern is even more evident. This pattern is characterized not only by an internal or intrapsychic chronic preoccupation with abandonment, but also by certain forms of behavior directed toward others—for example, angry demandingness—which has interpersonal consequences, including increasing the risk of bringing about the very abandonment that is also deeply feared.[3] It seems to me that attachment research on the interactive

---

[3]In the psychoanalytic context, what one might call the interpersonalization of defense is seen in the currently popular concept of projective identification, as elaborated by Ogden (1982). On that view, individual A not only projects an unacceptable wish or aspect of himself or herself to the individual B—which could remain at a purely intrapsychic level—but also *induces* individual B to feel and act in a certain way. Hence, an intrapsychic defense is transformed to include an interpersonal aspect. It is interesting to observe that of all the defenses formulated by Freud and Anna Freud, it is projection that is directed outward and that is inherently interpersonal, or using contemporary language, two-person rather than one-person. That is, one projects something about oneself onto another person and then experiences as well as relates to that person in a different way.

context and interpersonal consequences of different attachment patterns can enrich the psychoanalytic concept of defense.

CONCLUDING COMMENTS

To what extent can attachment research and theory and psychoanalytic theories be integrated? There are two possibilities. One is the current state of affairs characterized by two different theories, different domains, different traditions, different methods, and different sources of data, with interesting connections between them. The other possibility lies in attempts at integration of the kinds of phenomena and data that I have described into attachment theory and research. For example, the concept of an internal working model can be expanded to include such phenomena as "devotion" and "obstinate attachment" to early objects and guilt-motivated unconscious pathogenic beliefs identified in psychoanalytic theory.

Of course, one can start with the phenomena and data that are identified by attachment theory and research and ask whether they can be integrated into psychoanalytic theory. The latter seems a more difficult task because, in contrast to the relatively unified status of attachment theory, we know what its core tenets and propositions are—psychoanalytic theory is characterized by different "schools" and little consensus on core tenets and propositions.

One of the most fruitful potential consequences of a greater integration between attachment theory and research and psychoanalysis is the exploration, fleshing out, and testing, in a language susceptible to empirical investigation and to interdisciplinary integration, the implications of psychoanalytic formulations. To a certain extent, this has already been done. For example, Fairbairn's (1952) claim that "libido is object-seeking" or Balint's (1937/1965) concept of "primary object love" can be embedded in a broad evolutionary and empirically grounded context. This is also the case for more recent psychoanalytic concepts and formulations. For example, Mitchell (1988) writes that from the perspective of relational psychoanalysis, mind is made up of "relational configurations" (p. 3) (rather than a "cauldron full of seething excitations" [Freud, p. 84]). One can think of Bowlby's concept of the internal working model and many of the research findings on attachment patterns as "fleshing out" this view of the mind. This is not simply a matter of translation. Rather, it is a matter of giving these concepts empirical reference and embedding them in an accompanying research program.

In doing the necessary thinking, reading, and research in writing this book, I have been struck by a clear contrast between attachment and psychoanalytic theories in their respective practices, values, and attitudes, particularly in regard to how each discipline goes about developing knowledge, constructing theory, and resolving conflicting hypotheses and formulations. It is, of course, true that insofar as psychoanalysis is also a form of treatment, one would expect certain differences with regard to goals and practices. However, insofar as psychoanalysis is also a *theory*, (Indeed, Strachey [1937, p. 212] suggests that Freud "was always eager to direct attention to the importance of the non-therapeutic interests of psychoanalysis, the direction in which lay his own personal preferences, particularly in the later part of his life."), the issue of clinical focus cannot account for all the differences in practices, values, and attitudes between attachment and psychoanalytic theories.

I was particularly struck by the differences between the two disciplines in reviewing the perplexing issue of the relationship between maternal sensitivity and infant attachment status. Let me re-trace that issue as a means of highlighting the contrast between the practices of attachment and psychoanalytic theories. As noted, according to attachment theory, there should be a robust relationship between the two—a finding reported by Ainsworth et al. (1978). And yet, that robust relationship did not appear to be generally found. How can one account for that? One possibility, as we have seen, is that maternal sensitivity was not adequately measured. And, indeed, the more the measurement of maternal sensitivity resembled the Ainsworth et al. (1978) assessment, the stronger the relationship between maternal sensitivity and infant attachment status (De Wolff & van IJzendoorn, 1997). However, in no study reviewed in De Wolff and van IJzendoorn's meta-analysis was the relationship between maternal sensitivity and infant attachment as strong as that reported by Ainsworth et al. (1978).

Further progress in shedding light on the issue is provided by three additional sets of findings: One, because maternal behaviors other than sensitivity influence the child's development, including his or her attachment status, one should perhaps not expect as strong a relationship between sensitivity and attachment as originally proposed. Two, contextual factors, such as socioeconomic status and family conflict, moderate the influence of maternal sensitivity. And three, and especially interesting and provocative, is the finding that genetically based individual differences in susceptibility to rearing influences appear to moderate the effects of maternal behaviors on the child's development, including his or her attachment status. In short, there is a systematic effort, based on empirical evidence, to clarify a puzzling and complex issue in a piecemeal and cumulative way.

Contrastingly, in the psychoanalytic context, theoretical claims, for example, on the relationship between early experiences and later development, are often based on authoritative generalizations from clinical experience with one or two cases. Freud's universalization of findings from single cases set a precedent for this practice. Also, as we have seen, theoretical generalizations are almost always based on "follow-back" data from patients in treatment, which paints a misleading etiological picture. And finally, there is little effort to modify claims through systematic empirical investigation. Rather, different theoretical claims are presented in the context of competing "schools" associated with the formulations of charismatic leaders.

Perhaps, then, the most important general contribution attachment theory and research can make to psychoanalysis is providing a model for integrating clinical and theoretical concepts and formulations with a broad empirical research program. They can also serve as a model for theory building and for adjudicating debates on clinical and theoretical questions on the basis of careful conceptual analysis and empirical data rather than citations of presumably authoritative authors accompanied by selective clinical vignettes. Finally, the history of attachment theory can also serve as a model for an openness to formulations and findings from other disciplines.

References

Abrams, K., Rifkin, A., & Hesse, E. (2006). Examining the role of parental frightened/frightening subtypes in predicting disorganized attachment within a brief observation procedure. *Development and Psychopathology, 18*, 345–361.

Adam, E. K., Sheldon-Keller, A. E., & West, M. (1996). Attachment organization and history of suicidal behavior in clinical adolescents. *Journal of Consulting and Clinical Psychology, 64*, 264–272.

Agrawal, H. R., Gunderson, J., Holmes, B. M., & Lyons-Ruth, K. (2004). Attachment studies with borderline patients: A review. *Harvard Review of Psychiatry, 12*(2), 94–104.

Aguilar, B., Sroufe, L. A., Egeland, B., & Carlson, E. (2000). Distinguishing the early-onset/persistent and adolescence-onset antisocial behavior types: From birth to 16 years. *Development and Psychopathology, 12*, 109–132.

Ainsworth, M. D. S. (1967). *Infancy in Uganda: Infant care and the growth of attachment*. Baltimore: Johns Hopkins University Press.

Ainsworth, M. D. S., Bell, S. M., & Stayton, D. J. (1974). Infant–mother attachment and social development: "Socialization" as a product of reciprocal responsiveness to signals. In M. P. M. Richards (Ed.), *The integration of a child with a social world* (pp. 99–135). New York: Cambridge University Press.

Ainsworth, M. D. S., Blehar, M. C., Waters, E., & Wall, S. (1978). *Patterns of attachment: A psychological study of the Strange Situation*. Hillsdale, NJ: Erlbaum.

Allen, E. S., & Baucom, D. H. (2004). Adult attachment and patterns of extradyadic involvement. *Family Process, 43*, 467–488.

Allen, J. G., Fonagy, P., & Bateman, A. W. (2008). *Mentalizing in clinical practice*. Washington, DC: American Psychiatric Publishing.

Allen, J. P., Porter, M., McFarland, C., McElhaney, K., & Marsh, P. (2007). The relation of attachment security to adolescents' paternal and peer relationships, depression, and externalizing behavior. *Child Development*, *78*(4), 1222–1239.

Ammaniti, M., Speranza, A., & Fedele, S. (2005). Attachment in infancy and in early and late childhood: A longitudinal study. In K. A. Kerns & R. A. Richardson (Eds.), *Attachment in middle childhood* (pp. 115–136). New York: Guilford Press.

Anisfeld, E., Casper, V., Nozyce, M., & Cunningham, N. (1990). Does infant carrying promote attachment?: An experimental study of the effects of increased physical contact on the development of attachment. *Child Development*, *61*(5), 1617–1627.

Aviezer, O., Sagi, A., Resnick, G., & Gini, M. (2002). School competence in young adolescence: Links to early attachment relationships beyond concurrent self-perceived competence and representations of relationships. *International Journal of Behavioral Development*, *26*(5), 397–409.

Babcock, J. C., Jacobson, N. S., Gottman, J. M., & Yerington, T. P. (2000). Attachment, emotional regulation, and the function of marital violence: Differences between secure, preoccupied, and dismissing violent and nonviolent husbands. *Journal of Family Violence*, *15*, 391–409.

Bacciagaluppi, M. (1994). The influence of Ferenczi on Bowlby. *International Forum of Psychoanalysis*, *3*(2), 97–101.

Bachelor, A., Meunier, G., Laverdiére, O., & Gamache, D. (2010). Client attachment to therapist: Relation to client personality and symptomatology, and their contributions to the therapeutic alliance. *Psychotherapy: Theory, Research, Practice, Training*, *47*(4), 454–468.

Bakermans-Kranenburg, M. J., van IJzendoorn, M. H., & Juffer, F. (2003). Less is more: Meta-analyses of sensitivity and attachment interventions in early childhood. *Psychological Bulletin*, *129*, 195–215.

Bakermans-Kranenburg, M. J., van IJzendoorn, M. H., & Juffer, F. (2005). Disorganized infant attachment and preventive interventions: A review and meta-analysis. *Infant Mental Health Journal*, *26*, 191–216.

Bakermans-Kranenburg, M. J., van IJzendoorn, M. H., Mesman, J., Alink, L., & Juffer, F. (2008). Effects of an attachment-based intervention on daily cortisol moderated by dopamine receptor D4: A randomized control trial on 1- to 3-year-olds screened for externalizing behavior. *Development and Psychopathology*, *20*(3), 805–820.

Bakermans-Kranenburg, M. J., van IJzendoorn, M. H., Pijlman, F. A., Mesman, J., & Juffer, F. (2008). Experimental evidence for differential susceptibility: Dopamine D4 receptor polymorphism (DRD4 VNTR) moderates intervention effects on toddlers' externalizing behavior in a randomized controlled trial. *Developmental Psychology*, *44*(1), 293–300.

Balint, M. (1937). Early developmental styles of the ego: Primary object love. In *Primary love and psychoanalytic technique* (pp. 234–267). New York: Liveright, 1965.

Balint, M. (1949). Early developmental states of the ego: Primary object love. *International Journal of Psycho-Analysis*, *30*, 265–273.

Barnard, C. J., & Aldhous, P. (1991). Kinship, kin discrimination and mate choice.

In P. G. Hepper (Ed.), *Kin recognition* (pp. 125–147). Cambridge, UK: Cambridge University Press.

Barnard, C. J., & Fitzsimons, J. (1988). Kin recognition and mate choice in mice: The effects of kinship familiarity and social interference on intersexual interactions. *Animal Behaviour, 36,* 1078–1090.

Barnard, K. E. (1998). Developing, implanting, and documenting interventions with parents and young children. *Zero to Three, 18*(4), 23–29.

Barnard, K. E., Magyary, D., Summer, G., Booth, C. L., Mitchell, S. K., & Spieker, S. (1988). Prevention of parenting alterations for women with low social support. *Psychiatry, 51,* 248–253.

Barnard, K. E., Morisset, C., & Spieker, S. (1993). Preventive interventions: Enhancing parent–infant relationships. In C. H. Zeanah (Ed.), *Handbook of infant mental health* (pp. 386–401). New York: Guilford Press.

Barnett, B., Blignault, I., Holmes, S., Payne, A., & Parker, G. (1987). Quality of attachment in a sample of 1-year-old Australian children. *Journal of the American Academy of Child and Adolescent Psychiatry, 26*(3), 303–307.

Barone, L. (2003). Developmental protective and risk factors in borderline personality disorder: A study using the adult attachment interview. *Attachment and Human Development, 5,* 64–77.

Barr, G. A., Moriceau, S., Shionoya, K., Muzny, K., Gao, P., Wang, S., et al. (2009). Transitions in infant learning are modulated by dopamine in the amygdala. *Nature Neuroscience, 12,* 1367–1369.

Bartholomew, K., & Allison, C. J. (2006). An attachment perspective on abusive dynamics in intimate relationships. In M. Mikulincer & G. S. Goodman (Eds.), *Dynamics of romantic love: Attachment, caregiving, and sex* (pp. 102–127). New York: Guilford Press.

Bateman, A., & Fonagy, P. (2001). Treatment of borderline personality disorder with psychoanalytically oriented partial hospitalization: An 18-month follow-up. *American Journal of Psychiatry, 158*(1), 36–42.

Bateman, A., & Fonagy, P. (2006). *Mentalization-based treatment for borderline personality disorder.* New York: Oxford University Press.

Bateson, P. (1983). Optimal outbreeding. In P. Bateson (Ed.), *Mate choice* (pp. 257–277). Cambridge, UK: Cambridge University Press.

Bateson, P. P. G. (1982). Preferences for cousins in Japanese quail. *Nature, 295,* 236–237.

Beebe, B., Jaffe, J., Markese, S., Buck, K., Chen, H., Cohen, P., et al. (2010). The origins of 12-month attachment: A microanalysis of 4-month mother–infant interaction. *Attachment and Human Development, 12*(1/2), 3–141.

Beebe, B., & Lachmann, F. (1994). Representation and internalization in infancy: Three principles of salience. *Psychoanalytic Psychology, 11,* 127–165.

Beebe, B., & Lachmann, F. (2002). *Infant research and adult treatment: Co-constructing interactions.* Hillsdale, NJ: Analytic Press.

Belsky, J. (1997a). Theory testing, effect-size evaluation, and differential susceptibility to rearing influence: The case of mothering and attachment. *Child Development, 64,* 598–600.

Belsky, J. (1997b). Variation in susceptibility to environmental influence: An evolutionary argument. *Psychological Inquiry, 8,* 182–186.

Belsky, J. (2005). Differential susceptibility to rearing influence: An evolutionary hypothesis and some evidence. In B. Ellis & D. Bjorklund (Eds.), *Origins of the social mind: Evolutionary psychology and child development* (pp. 139–163). New York: Guilford Press.

Belsky, J., Bakermans-Kranenburg, M. J., & van IJzendoorn, M. H. (2007). For better *and* for worse: Differential susceptibility to environmental influences. *Current Directions in Psychological Science, 16,* 300–304.

Belsky, J., & Fearon, R. (2002). Early attachment security, subsequent maternal sensitivity, and later child development: Does continuity in development depend upon continuity of caregiving? *Attachment and Human Development, 4*(3), 361–387.

Belsky, J., Hsieh, K., & Crnic, K. (1998). Mothering, fathering, and infant negativity as antecedents of boys' externalizing problems and inhibition at age 3 years: Differential susceptibility to rearing experience? *Development and Psychopathology, 10,* 301–319.

Berant, E., Mikulincer, M., Shaver, P. R., & Segal, Y. (2005). Rorschach correlates of self-reported attachment dimensions: Dynamic manifestations of hyperactivating and deactivating strategies. *Journal of Personality Assessment, 84*(1), 70–81.

Bereczkei, T., Gyuris, P., Koves, P., & Bernath, L. (2002). Homogamy, genetic similarity, and imprinting: Parental influence on mate choice preferences. *Personality and Individual Differences, 33,* 677–690.

Berlin, L. J. (2005). Interventions to enhance early attachments: The state of the field today. In L. J. Berlin, Y. Ziv, L. Amaya-Jackson, & M. T. Greenberg (Eds.), *Enhancing early attachments: Theory, research, interventions, and policy* (pp. 3–33). New York: Guilford Press.

Berlin, L. J., Zeanah, C. H., & Lieberman, A. F. (2008). Prevention and intervention programs for supporting early attachment security. In J. Cassidy & P. R. Shaver (Eds.), *Handbook of attachment: Theory, research, and clinical applications* (2nd ed., pp. 745–761). New York: Guilford Press.

Bermant, G. (1976). Sexual behaviour: Hard times with the Coolidge effect. In M. H. Siegel & H. P. Zeigler (Eds.), *Psychological research: The inside story.* New York: Harper & Row.

Bernier, A., Larose, S., & Whipple, N. (2005). Leaving home for college: A potentially stressful event for adolescents with preoccupied attachment patterns. *Attachment and Human Development, 7*(2), 171–185.

Black, M. (1967). Review of A. R. Couch's "Explanation and human action." *American Journal of Psychology, 80,* 655–656.

Blatt, S. T. (2004). *Experiences of depression: Treatment, clinical, and research perspectives.* Washington, DC: American Psychological Association.

Block, J. (1978). *The Q-sort method in personality assessment and psychiatric research.* Palo Alto, CA: Consulting Psychologists Press. (Original work published 1961)

Blumstein, P., & Schwartz, P. (1983). *American couples.* New York: Morrow.

Bogaert, A. F., & Sadava, S. (2002). Adult attachment and sexual behavior. *Personal Relationships, 9*, 191–204.

Bosquet, M., & Egeland, B. (2006). The development and maintenance of anxiety symptoms from infancy through adolescence in a longitudinal sample. *Development and Psychopathology, 18*, 517–550.

Bowlby, J. (1944). Forty-four juvenile thieves: Their characters and home life. *International Journal of Psychoanalysis, 25*, 19–52.

Bowlby, J. (1958). The nature of the child's ties to his mother. *International Journal of Psychoanalysis, 39*, 350–373.

Bowlby, J. (1960). Grief and mourning in infancy and early childhood. *Psychoanalytic Study of the Child, 15*, 9–52.

Bowlby, J. (1969). *Attachment and loss: Vol. 1. Attachment.* New York: Basic Books, 1982.

Bowlby, J. (1973). *Attachment and loss: Vol. 2. Separation: Anxiety and anger.* New York: Basic Books.

Bowlby, J. (1979). *The making and breaking of affectional bonds.* London: Tavistock.

Bowlby, J. (1980). *Attachment and loss: Vol. 3. Loss: Sadness and depression.* London: Hogarth Press and Institute of Psycho-Analysis.

Bowlby, J. (1988). *A secure base: Clinical applications of attachment theory.* London: Routledge.

Brennan, K. A., Clark, C. L., & Shaver, P. R. (1998). Self-report measurement of adult attachment: An integrative overview. In J. A. Simpson & W. S. Rholes (Eds.), *Attachment theory and close relationships* (pp. 46–76). New York: Guilford Press.

Bretherton, I. (1987). New perspectives on attachment relations: Security, communication, and internal working models. In J. Osofsky (Eds.), *Handbook of infant development* (2nd ed., pp. 1061–1100). Oxford, UK: Wiley.

Bretherton, I. (1990). Communication patterns, internal working models, and the intergenerational transmission of attachment relationships. *Infant Mental Health Journal, 11*(3), 237–252.

Bretherton, I., Prentiss, C., & Ridgeway, D. (1990). Family relationships as represented in a story-completion task at thirty-seven and fifty-four months of age. *New Directions for Child Development, 48*, 85–105.

Brisch, K. H. (2002). *Treating attachment disorders: From theory to therapy.* New York: Guilford Press.

Brisch, K. H. (2012). *Treating attachment disorders: From theory to therapy* (2nd ed.). New York: Guilford Press.

Bromberg, P. (1996). *Standing in the spaces.* Hillsdale, NJ: Analytic Press.

Brussoni, M. J., Jeng, K. L., Livesley, W. J., & MacBeth, T. M. (2000). Genetic and environmental influences on adult attachment styles. *Personal Relationships, 7*, 283–289.

Bucci, W. (1997). *Psychoanalysis and cognitive science.* New York: Guilford Press.

Buchheim, A., Heinrichs, M., George, C., Pokorny, D., Koops, E., Henningsen, P., et al. (2009). Oxytocin enhances the experience of attachment security. *Psychoneuroendocrinology, 34*, 1417–1422.

Burlingham, D. T., & Freud, A. (1944). *Infants without families*. New York: International Universities Press.

Busch, F. (2009). On creating a psychoanalytic mind: Psychoanalytic knowledge as a process. *Scandinavian Psychoanalytic Review, 32*, 85–92.

Byng-Hall, J. (1995). *Rewriting family scripts*. New York: Guilford Press.

Byng-Hall, J. (1998). Evolving ideas about narrative: Re-editing the re-editing of family mythology. *Journal of Family Therapy, 20*, 133–141.

Carlson, E. A. (1998). A prospective longitudinal study of attachment disorganization/disorientation. *Child Development, 69*(4), 1107.

Carlson, V., Cicchetti, D., Barnett, D., & Braunwald, K. (1989). Disorganized/disoriented attachment relationships in maltreated infants. *Developmental Psychology, 25*(4), 525–531.

Carnelley, K. B., Pietromonaco, P. R., & Jaffe, K. (1994). Depression, working models of others and relationship functioning. *Journal of Personality and Social Psychology, 66*, 127–140.

Cassidy, J., & Berlin, L. J. (1994). The insecure/ambivalent pattern of attachment: Theory and research. *Child Development, 65*, 971–981.

Cassidy, J., & Marvin, R. (1992). *Attachment organization in preschool children: Procedures and coding manual*. Unpublished manuscript, Pennsylvania State University and University of Virginia.

Cassidy, J., & Shaver, P. R. (Eds.). (2008). *Handbook of attachment: Theory, research, and clinical applications* (2nd ed.). New York: Guilford Press.

Cicchetti, D., Rogosch, F. A., & Toth, S. L. (2006). Fostering secure attachment in infants in maltreating families through preventive interventions. *Development and Psychopathology, 18*, 623–650.

Ciechanowski, P. S., Katon, W. J., & Hirsch, I. B. (2002). Interpersonal predictors of HbA_{1c} in patients with type 1 diabetes. *Diabetes Care, 25*(4), 731.

Clarke, G. (2011). Suttie's influence on Fairbairn's object relations theory. *Journal of the American Psychoanalytic Association, 59*(5), 939–960.

Coan, J. A., Schaefer, H. S., & Davidson, R. J. (2006). Lending a hand: Social regulation of the neural response to threat. *Psychological Science, 17*(12), 1032–1039.

Cohen, A. B. (2005). The relation of attachment to infidelity in romantic relationships: An exploration of attachment style, perception of partner's attachment style, relationship satisfaction, relationship quality and gender differences in sexual behaviors (doctoral dissertation, Adelphi University, The Institute of Advanced Psychological Studies). *ProQuest Dissertations and Theses*, Publication No. 3213084.

Cohen, J. (1988). *Statistical power analysis for the behavioral sciences* (new ed.). New York: Academic Press.

Cole-Detke, H., & Kobak, R. (1996). Attachment processes in eating disorder and depression. *Journal of Consulting and Clinical Psychology, 64*(2), 282–290.

Collins, N. L., & Read, S. J. (1990). Adult attachment, working models, and relationship quality in dating couples. *Journal of Personality and Social Psychology, 58*(4), 644–663.

Craik, K. (1943). *The nature of explanation*. Cambridge, UK: Cambridge University Press.

Cramer, P., & Eagle, M. (1972). Relationship between conditions of CRS representation and the category of false recognition. *Journal of Experimental Psychology, 94*, 1–5.

Creasey, G., & Ladd, A. (2005). Generalized and specific attachment representations: Unique and interactive roles in predicting conflict behaviors in close relationships. *Society for Personality and Social Psychology Bulletin, 31*(8), 1026–1038.

Critchfield, K., Levy, K., Clarkin, J., & Kernberg, O. (2008). The relational context of aggression in borderline personality disorder: Using adult attachment style to predict forms of hostility. *Journal of Clinical Psychology, 64*(1), 67–82.

Crittenden, P. M. (1994). Peering into the black box: An exploratory treatise on the development of the self in young children. In D. Cicchetti & S. Toth (Eds.), *Rochester Symposium on Developmental Psychopathology: The self and its disorders* (pp. 79–148). Rochester, NY: University of Rochester Press.

Crowell, J. A., Treboux, D., Gao, Y., Fyffe, C., Pan, H., & Waters, E. (2002). Assessing secure base behavior in adulthood: Development of a measure, links to adult attachment representations, and relations to couples' communication and reports of relationships. *Developmental Psychology, 38*(5), 679.

Crowell, J. A., Treboux, D., & Waters, E. (1999). The Adult Attachment Interview and the Relationship Questionnaire: Relations to reports of mothers and partners. *Personal Relationships, 6*, 1–18.

Davis, D., Follette, W. C., & Vernon, M. L. (2001, May). *Adult attachment style and the experience of unwanted sex*. Maui, HI: Western Psychological Association.

Davis, D., Shaver, P. R., & Vernon, M. L. (2004). Attachment style and subjective motivations for sex. *Personality and Social Psychology Bulletin, 30*, 1076–1090.

Davis, L. V., & Carlson, B. E. (1987). Observation of spouse abuse: What happens to the children? *Journal of Interpersonal Violence, 2*(3), 278–291.

DeKlyen, M., & Greenberg, M. T. (2008). Attachment and psychopathology in childhood. In J. Cassidy & P. R. Shaver (Eds.), *Handbook of attachment: Theory, research and clinical applications* (2nd ed., pp. 637–666). New York: Guilford Press.

Dennett, D. C. (1987). *The intentional stance*. Cambridge, MA: MIT Press.

De Wolff, M. S., & van IJzendoorn, M. H. (1997). Sensitivity and attachment: A meta-analysis on parental antecedents of infant attachment. *Child Development, 68*, 571–591.

Diamond, D., Stovall-McClough, C., Clarkin, J. F., & Levy, K. N. (2003). Patient–therapist attachment in the treatment of borderline personality disorder. *Bulletin of the Menninger Clinic, 67*, 227–259.

Diamond, J. (1992). *The third chimpanzee: The evolution and future of the human animal*. New York: HarperCollins.

Diamond, L. M. (2003). What does sexual orientation orient?: A biobehavioral model distinguishing romantic love and sexual desire. *Psychological Review*, *110*, 173–192.

Dodge, K. A., Pettit, G. S., Bates, J. E., & Valente, E. (1995). Social information processing patterns partially mediate the effect of early abuse on later conduct problems. *Journal of Abnormal Psychology*, *104*, 632–643.

Dollard, J., & Miller, N. E. (1950). *Personality and psychotherapy*. New York: McGraw-Hill.

Doumas, D. M., Pearson, C. L., Elgin, J. E., & McKinley, L. L. (2008). Adult attachment as a risk factor for intimate partner violence: The "mispairing" of partners' attachment styles. *Journal of Interpersonal Violence*, *23*, 616–634.

Dozier, M., Chase Stovall-McClough, K., & Albus, K. E. (2008). Attachment and psychopathology in adulthood. In J. Cassidy & P. R. Shaver (Eds.), *Handbook of attachment: Theory, research, and clinical applications* (2nd ed., pp. 718–744). New York: Guilford Press.

Dozier, M., Cue, K., & Barnett, L. (1994). Clinicians as caregivers: Role of attachment organization in treatment. *Journal of Consulting and Clinical Psychology*, *62*, 793–800.

Dozier, M., & Kobak, R. R. (1992). Psychophysiology in Adult Attachment Interviews: Converging evidence for de-activating strategies. *Child Development*, *63*, 1473–1480.

Dutra, L., & Lyons-Ruth, K. (2005). *Maltreatment, maternal and child psychopathology, and quality of early care as predictors of adolescent dissociation*. Paper presented at the biennial meeting of the Society for Research in Child Development, Atlanta, GA.

Eagle, M. N. (1962). Personality correlates of sensitivity to subliminal stimulation. *Journal of Nervous and Mental Disease*, *15*, 579–582.

Eagle, M. N. (1967). The effects of learning strategies upon free recall. *American Journal of Psychology*, *80*, 421–425.

Eagle, M. N. (1982). Essay review of J. Bowlby's *Loss: Attachment and loss, Vol. 3*. *Review of Psychoanalytic Books*, *1*, 57–64.

Eagle, M. N. (1987). The psychoanalytic and the cognitive unconscious. In R. Stern (Ed.), *Theories of the unconscious and theories of the self* (pp. 155–189). Hillsdale, NJ: Analytic Press.

Eagle, M. N. (1995). The developmental perspectives of attachment and psychoanalytic theory. In S. Goldberg, R. Muir, & J. Kerr (Eds.), *Attachment theory: Social, developmental and clinical perspectives* (pp. 123–150). Hillsdale, NJ: Analytic Press.

Eagle, M. N. (1996). Attachment research and psychoanalytic theory. In J. M. Masling & R. F. Bornstein (Eds.), *Psychoanalytic perspectives on developmental psychology*. Washington, DC: American Psychological Association.

Eagle, M. N. (1997). Attachment and psychoanalysis. *British Journal of Medical Psychology*, *70*, 217–229.

Eagle, M. N. (2006). Attachment, psychopathology, and assessment: A commentary. *Journal of Consulting and Clinical Psychology*, *74*, 1086–1097.

Eagle, M. N. (2007). Attachment and sexuality. In D. Diamond, S. Blatt, & J.

Lichtenberg (Eds.), *Attachment and sexuality* (pp. 27–50). New York: Analytic Press.

Eagle, M. N., & Cox-Steiner, G. (Eds.). (2001). Attachment: Current research, theory, and clinical practice. *Journal of Infant and Adolescent Psychotherapy* (Whole Issue).

Eagle, M. N., & Hill, A. L. (1969). Do disappearance patterns in low illumination constitute a perceptual phenomenon or a response artifact? *Nature, 224,* 282.

Eagle, M. N., & Leiter, E. (1964). Recall and recognition in intentional and incidental learning. *Journal of Experimental Psychology, 66,* 58–63.

Eagle, M. N., & Mulliken, S. (1974). The effect of affective ratings upon intentional and incidental learning. *American Journal of Psychology, 87,* 409–423.

Eagle, M. N., & Ortof, E. (1967). The effects of levels of attention upon "phonetic" recognition errors. *Journal of Verbal Learning and Verbal Behavior, 6,* 226–231.

Eagle, M. N., & Wolitzky, D. L. (2011). Systematic empirical research versus clinical case studies: A valid antagonism? *Journal of the American Psychoanalytic Association, 59,* 791–817.

Eagle, M. N., Wolitzky, D. L., & Klein, G. S. (1966). Imagery: Effect of a concealed figure in a stimulus. *Science, 151,* 837–839.

Eagle, M. N., Wolitzky, D. L., & Wakefield, J. C. (2001). The analyst's knowledge and authority: A critique of the "New View" in psychoanalysis. *Journal of the American Psychoanalytic Association, 49,* 457–488.

Eagle, R. S. (1990). Denial of access: Past, present, and future. *Canadian Psychology, 31,* 121–131.

Eagle, R. S. (1993). Airplanes crash, spaceships stay in orbit: The separation experience of a child "in care." *Journal of Psychotherapy: Research and Practice, 2,* 318–333.

Eagle, R. S. (1994). The separation experience of children in long-term care: Theory, resources, and implications for practice. *American Journal of Orthopsychiatry, 64,* 421–434.

Eames, V., & Roth, A. (2000). Patient attachment orientation and the early working alliance: A study of patient and therapist reports of alliance quality and ruptures. *Psychotherapy Research, 10,* 421–434.

Edelstein, R. S., Chopik, W. T., & Kean, E. L. (2011). Sociosexuality moderates the association between testosterone and relationship status in men and women. *Hormones and Behavior, 60,* 248–255.

Egeland, B., Weinfield, N. S., Bosquet, M., & Cheng, V. K. (2000). Remember, repeating, and working through: Lessons from attachment-based interventions. In J. Osofsky & H. E. Fitzgerald (Eds.), *WAIMH handbook of infant mental health* (Vol. 4, pp. 35–89). New York: Wiley.

Endler, N. S., & Magnusson, D. (1976). Toward an interactional psychology of personality. *Psychological Bulletin, 83*(5), 956–974.

Fairbairn, W. D. (1952). *Psychoanalytic studies of the personality.* London: Tavistock.

Farrugia, C., & Hogans, L. (1998, November 25–27). *Conceptualizing the pain bond: Attachment, caregiving, and sexuality as predictors of intimacy in adult romantic relationships.* Paper presented at the Sixth Australian Institute of Family Studies Conference, Melbourne, Australia.

Feeney, J. A., & Noller, P. (1990). Attachment style as a predictor of adult romantic relationships. *Journal of Personality and Social Psychology, 58*, 281–291.

Ferenczi, S. (1933). The confusion of tongues between adults and children: The language of tenderness and passion. In M. Balint (Ed.), *Final contributions to the problems and methods of psychoanalysis* (Vol. III, pp. 156–167). New York: Basic Books, 1955.

Finkel, D., Wille, D., & Matheny, A. (1998). Preliminary results from a twin study of infant–caregiver attachment. *Behavior Genetics, 28*(1), 1–8.

Finnegan, R. A., Hodges, E. V. E., & Perry, D. G. (1996). Preoccupied and avoidant coping during middle childhood. *Child Development, 67*, 1318–1328.

Finzi, R., Ram, A., Har-Even, D., Shnit, D., & Weizman, A. (2001). Attachment styles and aggression in physically abused and neglected children. *Journal of Youth and Adolescence, 30*(6), 769–786.

Fisher, H. E. (1998). Lust, attraction, and attachment in mammalian reproduction. *Human Nature, 9*, 23–52.

Fisher, H. E. (2000). Lust, attraction, and attachment. *Journal of Sex Education and Therapy, 25*, 96–104.

Fonagy, P. (1997). Attachment and theory of mind: Overlapping constructs? *Association for Child Psychology and Psychiatry Occasional Papers, 14*, 31–40.

Fonagy, P. (1999). Male perpetrators of violence against women: An attachment theory perspective. *Journal of Applied Psychoanalytic Studies, 1*, 7–27.

Fonagy, P. (2001). *Attachment theory and psychoanalysis.* New York: Other Press.

Fonagy, P., Bateman, A. W., & Luyten, P. (2012). Introduction and overview. In A. W. Bateman & P. Fonagy (Eds.), *Handbook of mentalizing in mental health practice* (pp. 3–42). Washington, DC: American Psychiatric Publishing.

Fonagy, P., Leigh, T., Steele, M., Steele, H., Kennedy, R., Mattoon, G., et al. (1996). The relation of attachment status, psychiatric classification, and response to psychotherapy. *Journal of Consulting and Clinical Psychology, 64*, 22–31.

Fonagy, P., Steele, H., & Steele, M. (1991). Maternal representations of attachment during pregnancy predict the organization of infant mother attachment at one-year of age. *Child Development, 62*, 891–905.

Fonagy, P., Steele, M., Steele, H., Leigh, T., Kennedy, R., Mattoon, G., et al. (1995). Attachment, the reflective self, and borderline states. In S. Goldberg & J. Kerr (Eds.), *Attachment research: The state of the art* (pp. 233–278). New York: Analytic Press.

Fosha, D. (2000). *The transforming power of affect: A model of accelerated change.* New York: Basic Books.

Fox, R. (1980). *The red lamp of incest: What the taboo can tell us about who we are and how we got that way.* New York: Dutton.

Fraiberg, S. (1980). *Clinical studies in infant mental health: The first year of life.* London: Tavistock.

Fraiberg, S., Adelson, E., & Shapiro, V. (1975). Ghosts in the nursery: A psychoanalytic approach to the problems of impaired infant–mother relationships. *Journal of the American Academy of Child Psychiatry, 14,* 387–421.

Fraley, R., & Spieker, S. J. (2003). Are infant attachment patterns continuously or categorically distributed?: A taxometric analysis of strange situation behavior. *Developmental Psychology, 39*(3), 387–404.

Fraley, R. C., & Marks, M. J. (2010). Westermarck, Freud, and the incest taboo: Does familial resemblance activate sexual attraction? *Personality and Social Psychology Bulletin, 36,* 1202–1212.

Frankel, K. A., & Bates, J. E. (1990). Mother–toddler problem solving: Antecedents in attachment, home behavior, and temperament. *Child Development, 61,* 810–819.

Freud, A. (1960). Discussion of Dr. John Bowlby's paper. *Psychoanalytic Study of the Child, 15,* 53–62.

Freud, S. (1893). Some points for a comparative study of organic and hysterical motor paralysis. *Standard Edition,* Vol. 1, pp. 155–172. London: Hogarth Press, 1966.

Freud, S. (1900). The interpretation of dreams. *Standard Edition,* Vol. 4–5, pp. 1–627. London: Hogarth Press, 1953.

Freud, S. (1905). Three essays on the theory of sexuality. *Standard Edition,* Vol. 7, pp. 123–245. London: Hogarth Press, 1953.

Freud, S. (1912). On the universal tendency to debasement in the sphere of love (Contributions to the psychology of love II). *Standard Edition,* Vol. 11, pp. 177–190. London: Hogarth Press, 1957.

Freud, S. (1915a). A case of paranoia running counter to the psycho-analytic theory of the disease. *Standard Edition,* Vol. 14, pp. 261–272. London: Hogarth Press, 1963.

Freud, S. (1915b). Instincts and their vicissitudes. *Standard Edition,* Vol. 14, pp. 109–140. London: Hogarth Press, 1963.

Freud, S. (1915c). The unconscious. *Standard Edition,* Vol. 14, pp. 159–215. London: Hogarth Press, 1963.

Freud, S. (1916–1917). Introductory lectures on psycho-analysis. *Standard Edition,* Vol. 15–16, pp. 1–482. London: Hogarth Press, 1961.

Freud, S. (1918). From the history of an infantile neurosis. *Standard Edition,* Vol. 17, pp. 1–123. London: Hogarth Press, 1955.

Freud, S. (1920). The psychogenesis of a case of homosexuality in a woman. *Standard Edition,* Vol. 18, pp. 145–172. London: Hogarth Press, 1955.

Freud, S. (1924). The economic problem of masochism. *Standard Edition,* Vol. 19, pp. 155–170. London: Hogarth Press, 1961.

Freud, S. (1925a). An autobiographical study. *Standard Edition,* Vol. 20, pp. 1–74. London: Hogarth Press, 1959.

Freud, S. (1925b). Some psychical consequences of the anatomical distinction between the sexes. *Standard Edition,* Vol. 19, pp. 241–258. London: Hogarth Press, 1961.

Freud, S. (1926a). Inhibitions, symptoms and anxiety. *Standard Edition,* Vol. 20, pp. 75–175. London: Hogarth Press, 1959.

Freud, S. (1926b). The question of lay analysis. *Standard Edition*, Vol. 20, pp. 177–258. London: Hogarth Press, 1959.

Freud, S. (1931). Female sexuality. *Standard Edition*, Vol. 21, pp. 221–243. London: Hogarth Press, 1961.

Freud, S. (1933). New introductory lectures on psycho-analysis. *Standard Edition*, Vol. 22, pp. 1–182. London: Hogarth Press, 1964.

Freud, S. (1937a). Analysis terminable and interminable. *Standard Edition*, Vol. 23, pp. 209–253. London: Hogarth Press, 1964.

Freud, S. (1937b). Construction in analysis. *Standard Edition*, Vol. 23, pp. 255–269. London: Hogarth Press, 1964.

Freud, S. (1940). An outline of psycho-analysis. *Standard Edition*, Vol. 23, pp. 139–207. London: Hogarth Press, 1964.

Freud, S. (1950[1895]). Project for a scientific psychology. *Standard Edition*, Vol. 1. London: Hogarth Press.

Furman, W., Simon, V. A., & Shaffer, L. (2002). Adolescents' working models and styles for relationships with parents, friends, and romantic partners. *Child Development*, 73(1), 241–255.

Gabbard, G. O., & Horowitz, M. J. (2009). Insight, transference interpretation, and therapeutic change in the dynamic psychotherapy of borderline personality disorder. *American Journal of Psychiatry*, 166, 517–521.

Gaines, R. (1997). Detachment and continuity: The two tasks of mourning. *Contemporary Psychoanalysis*, 33(4), 549–571.

Gallo, L. C., & Matthews, K. A. (2006). Adolescent's attachment orientation influences ambulatory blood pressure responses to everyday social interaction. *Psychosomatic Medicine*, 68, 253–261.

Gergely, G. (1992). Developmental reconstructions: Infancy from the point of view of psychoanalysis and developmental psychology. *Psychoanalysis and Contemporary Thought*, 15(1), 3–55.

Gergely, G., & Unoka, Z. (2008). Attachment and mentalization in humans: The development of the affective self. In E. L. Jurist, A. Slade, & S. Bergner (Eds.), *Mind to mind: Infant research, neuroscience and psychoanalysis* (pp. 50–67). New York: Other Press.

Gervai, J., Novak, A., Lakatos, K., Toth, I., Danis, I., Ronal, Z., et al. (2007). Infant genotype may moderate sensitivity to maternal affective communications: Attachment disorganization, quality of care, and the DRD4 polymorphism. *Social Neuroscience*, 2, 1–13.

Gettler, L. T., Agustin, S. S., McDade, T. W., & Kuzawa, C. W. (2011). Short-term changes in fathers' hormones during father–child play: Impacts of paternal attitudes and experience. *Hormones and Behavior*, 60, 599–606.

Gillick, R. A., & Bone, S. (Eds.). (1990). *Pleasure beyond the pleasure principle*. New Haven, CT: Yale University Press.

Goldberg, S., Benoit, D., Blokland, K., & Madigan, S. (2003). Atypical maternal behavior, maternal representations, and infant disorganized attachment. *Development and Psychopathology*, 15, 239–257.

Gough, H. G., & Heilbrun, A. B. (1983). *The Adjective Checklist manual*. Palo Alto, CA: Consulting Psychologists Press.

Graham, C. A., & Easterbrooks, M. A. (2000). School-aged children's vulnerability to depressive symptomatology and economic risk. *Development and Psychopathology, 12,* 201–213.

Granot, D., & Mayseless, O. (2001). Attachment security and adjustment to school in middle childhood. *International Journal of Behavioral Development, 25*(6), 530–541.

Gray, P. (1994). *The ego and the analysis of defense.* Lanham, MD: Jason Aronson.

Green, A. (2000). Science and science fiction in infant research. In J. Sandler, A. M. Sandler, & R. Davies (Eds.), *Clinical and observational psychoanalytic research* (pp. 41–73). London: Karnac Books.

Greenberg, M. T. (2005). Enhancing early attachments: Synthesis and recommendations for research, practice, and policy. In L. G. Berlin, Y. Ziv, L. Amaya-Jackson, & M. T. Greenberg (Eds.), *Enhancing early attachments: Theory, research, interventions, and policy* (pp. 327–343). New York: Guilford Press.

Grienenberger, J., Kelly, K., & Slade, A. (2005). Maternal reflective functioning, mother–infant affective communication, and infant attachment: Exploring the link between mental states and observed caregiving behavior in the intergenerational transmission of attachment. *Attachment and Human Development, 7*(3), 299–311.

Grossman, L., & Eagle, M. (1970). Synonymity, antonymity, and association in false recognition. *Journal of Experimental Psychology, 83,* 244–248.

Grossmann, K. E., Grossmann, K., & Waters, E. (Eds.). (2005). *Attachment from infancy to adulthood: The major longitudinal studies.* New York: Guilford Press.

Gullestad, S. E. (2001). Attachment theory and psychoanalysis: Controversial issues. *Scandinavian Psychoanalytical Review, 24,* 3–16.

Gunderson, J. G., & Lyons-Ruth, K. (2008). BPD's interpersonal hypersensitivity phenotype: A gene–environment developmental model. *Journal of Personality Disorders, 22*(1), 22–41.

Hammen, C. L., Burge, D., Daley, S. E., & Davila, J. (1995). Interpersonal attachment cognitions and prediction of symptomatic responses to interpersonal stress. *Journal of Abnormal Psychology, 104*(3), 436–443.

Hardy, G. E., Aldridge, J., Davidson, C., Rowe, C., Reilly, S., & Shapiro, D. A. (1999). Therapist responsiveness to client attachment styles and issues observed in client-identified significant events in psychodynamic-interpersonal psychotherapy. *Psychotherapy Research, 9*(1), 36–53.

Harlow, H. F. (1958). The nature of love. *American Psychologist, 13,* 673–685.

Harlow, H. F. (1960). Primary affectional patterns in primates. *American Journal of Orthopsychiatry, 30,* 676–684.

Hartmann, H. (1958). *Ego psychology and the problem of adaptation* (D. Rapaport, Trans.). Madison, CT: International Universities Press.

Haydon, K. C., Roisman, G. I., & Burt, K. B. (2012). In search of security: The latent structure of the Adult Attachment Interview. *Development and Psychopathology, 24*(2), 589–606.

Haydon, K. C., Roisman, G. I., Marks, M. J., & Fraley, R. C. (2011). An empirically derived approach to the latent structure of the Adult Attachment Interview:

Additional convergent and discriminant validity evidence. *Attachment and Human Development, 13*(5), 503–524.

Hazan, C., & Shaver, P. R. (1987). Romantic love conceptualized as an attachment process. *Journal of Personality and Social Psychology, 52*, 511–524.

Hazan, C., & Zeifman, D. (1994). Sex and the psychological tether. In K. Bartholomew & D. Perlman (Eds.), *Advances in personal relationships: Vol. 5. Attachment processes in adulthood* (pp. 151–177). London: Jessica Kingsley.

Heinicke, C. M. (1956). *Some effects of separating two-year-old children from their parents: A comparative study.* London: Tavistock Institute of Human Relations.

Heinicke C., & Westheimer, I. (1966). *Brief separations.* New York: International Universities Press.

Heinrichs, M., Baumgartner, T., Kirschbaum, C., & Ehlert, U. (2003). Social support and oxytocin interact to suppress cortisol and subjective responses to psychosocial stress. *Biological Psychiatry 54*, 1389–1398.

Hendricks, I. (1943). The discussion of the "instinct to master." *Psychoanalytic Quarterly, 12*, 561–565.

Hermann, I. (1933). Zum Triebleben der Primaten [The instinctual life of primates]. *Imago, 19*, 113–125.

Hermann, I. (1936). Clinging and going-in-search. *Psychoanalytic Quarterly, 45*, 5–36.

Hesse, E., & Main, M. (2006). Frightened, threatening, and dissociative parental behavior in low-risk samples: Description, discussion, and interpretations. *Developmental Psychopathology, 18*, 309–343.

Hinde, R. A. (1982). *Ethology, its nature and relations with other sciences.* New York: Oxford University Press.

Hofer, M. A. (2006). Psychobiological roots of early attachment. *Current Directions in Psychological Science, 15*, 84–88.

Hofer, M. A. (1990). Early symbiotic processes: Hard evidence from a soft place. In R. A. Glick & S. Bone (Eds.), *Pleasure beyond the pleasure principle* (pp. 63–78). New Haven, CT: Yale University Press.

Hoffman, I. Z. (2009). Doublethinking our way to "scientific" legitimacy: The desiccation of human Schatzman experience. *Journal of the American Psychoanalytic Association, 57*, 1043–1069.

Hoffman, K. T., Marvin, R. S., Cooper, G., & Powell, B. (2006). Changing toddlers' and preschoolers' attachment classifications: The Circle of Security intervention. *Journal of Consulting and Clinical Psychology, 74*(6), 1017–1026.

Holmes, J. (1995). "Something there is that doesn't love a wall": John Bowlby, attachment theory, and psychoanalysis. In A. Muir & J. Kern (Eds.), *Attachment theory: Social, developmental, and clinical perspectives* (pp. 19–44). Hillsdale, NJ: Analytic Press.

Holmes, J. (2001). *The search for the secure base: Attachment theory and psychotherapy.* Hove, UK: Brunner-Routledge.

Holzworth-Munroe, A., Stuart, G. L., & Hutchinson, G. (1997). Violent versus nonviolent husbands: Differences in attachment patterns, dependency, and jealousy. *Journal of Family Psychology, 11*, 314–331.

Hughes, P., Turton, P., Hopper, E., McGauley, G., & Fonagy, P. (2001). Disorganized attachment behavior among infants born subsequent to stillbirth. *Journal of Child Psychology and Psychiatry and Allied Disciplines, 42*(6), 791–801.

Hull, C. L. (1943). *Principles of behavior: An introduction to behavior theory.* Oxford, UK: Appleton-Century.

Hull, C. L. (1951). *Essentials of behavior.* New Haven, CT: Yale University Press.

Huot, R. L., Plotsky, P. M., Lenox, R. H., & McNamara, R. K. (2002). Neonatal maternal separation reduces hippocampal mossy fiber density in adult Long–Evans rats. *Brain Research, 950*(1/2), 52–63.

Impett, E. A., & Peplau, L. A. (2002). Why some women consent to unwanted sex with a dating partner: Insights from attachment theory. *Psychology of Women Quarterly, 26*, 360–370.

Insel, T. R., & Young, L. J. (2001). The neurobiology of attachment. *Nature Reviews Neuroscience, 2*, 129–136.

Isaacs, S. (1943). The nature and function of phantasy. In R. Steven (Ed.), *Unconscious phantasy* (pp. 145–198). London: Karnac Books, 2003.

Isabella, R. A. (1993). Origins of attachment: Maternal interactive behavior across the first year. *Child Development, 64*, 605–621.

Israels, H., & Schatzman, M. (1993). The seduction theory. *History of Psychiatry, 4*, 23–59.

Jacobsen, T., Edelstein, W., & Hofmann, V. (1994). A longitudinal study of the relation between representations of attachment in childhood and cognitive functioning in childhood and adolescence. *Developmental Psychology, 30*, 112–124.

Jacobson, J. L., & Wille, D. E. (1986). The influence of attachment pattern on developmental changes in peer interaction from the toddler to the preschool period. *Child Development, 57*, 338–347.

Jacobvitz, D., & Hazan, N. (1999). Developmental pathways from infant disorganization to childhood peer relationships. In J. Solomon & C. George (Eds.), *Attachment disorganization* (pp. 127–159). New York: Guilford Press.

Jacobvitz, D., Leon, K., & Hazen, N. (2006). Does expectant mother's unresolved trauma predict frightened/frightening maternal behaviors?: Risk and protective factors. *Development and Psychopathology, 18*, 363–379.

Johnson, J. G., Cohen, P., Chen, H., Kasen, S., & Brook, J. S. (2006). Parenting behaviors associated with risk for offspring personality disorder during adulthood. *Archives of General Psychiatry, 63*, 579–587.

Johnson, S. M. (2008). Couple and family therapy: An attachment perspective. In J. Cassidy & P. R. Shaver (Eds.), *Handbook of attachment: Theory, research, and clinical applications* (2nd ed., pp. 811–829). New York: Guilford Press.

Jones, E. (1952). Foreword to Fairbairn's *Psychoanalytic studies of personality.* London: Tavistock.

Jurist, E. L., Slade, A., & Bergner, S. (2008). (Eds.). *Mind to mind: Infant research, neuroscience and psychoanalysis* (pp. 50–67). New York: Other Press.

Kagan, J. (1982). *Psychological research on the human infant: An evaluative summary.* New York: W. T. Grant Foundation.

Kagan, J. (1995). On attachment. *Harvard Review of Psychiatry, 3,* 104–106.

Karen, R. (1994). *Becoming attached: Unfolding the mystery of the infant–mother bond and its impact on later life.* New York: Warner Books.

Kazdin, A. E. (2001). Bridging the enormous gaps of theory with therapy research and practice. *Journal of Clinical and Child Psychology, 30*(1), 59–66.

Kernberg, O. F. (1976). *Object relations theory and clinical psychoanalysis.* New York: Jason Aronson.

Kernberg, O. F. (1980). *Internal world and external reality.* New York: Jason Aronson.

Kernberg, O. F. (1993). The psychopathology of hatred. In R. A. Gillick & S. P. Roose (Eds.), *Rage, power, and aggression: The role of affect in motivation, development, and adaptation.* (pp. 61–79). New Haven, CT: Yale University Press.

Kernberg, O. F. (1995). *Love relations: Normality and pathology.* New Haven, CT: Yale University Press.

Kernberg, O. F. (2005). Object relations theories and techniques. In E. Person, A. Cooper, & G. Gabbard (Eds.), *Textbook of psychoanalysis* (pp. 57–75). Washington, DC: American Psychiatric Publishing.

Kernberg, O. F., Yeomans, F. E., Clarkin, J. F., & Levy, K. N. (2008). Transference focused psychotherapy: Overview and update. *International Journal of Psychoanalysis, 89,* 601–620.

Kerns, K. A. (2008). Attachment in middle childhood. In J. Cassidy & P. R. Shaver (Eds.), *Handbook of attachment: Theory, research, and clinical applications* (2nd ed., pp. 366–382). New York: Guilford Press.

Kerns, K. A., Aspelmeier, J. E., Gentzler, A. L., & Grabill, C. M. (2001). Parent–child attachment and monitoring in middle childhood. *Journal of Family Psychology, 15*(1), 69–81.

Kilpatrick, K. L., & Williams, L. M. (1997). Post-traumatic stress disorder in child witnesses to intimate partner violence. *American Journal of Orthopsychiatry, 67,* 639–644.

Kinsey, A. C., Pomeroy, W. B., & Martin, C. E. (1948). *Sexual behavior in the human male.* Oxford, UK: Saunders.

Klein, G. S. (1976). Freud's two theories of sexuality. In M. M. Gill & P. S. Holzman (Eds.), *Psychology versus metapsychology: Psychoanalytic essays in memory of G. S. Klein* (pp. 14–70). New York: International Universities Press.

Klein, M. (1945). The Oedipus complex in the light of early anxieties. *International Journal of Psycho-Analysis, 26,* 11–33.

Klein, M. (1975). *Love, guilt and reparation and other works 1921–1945.* London: Hogarth Press.

Klein, M., Heimann, P., Isaacs, S., & Rivière, J. (1952). *Developments in psychoanalysis.* London: Hogarth Press.

Klerman, G. L., Weissman, M. M., Rounsaville, B. J., & Chevron, E. S. (1984). *Interpersonal psychotherapy for depression.* New York: Basic Books.

Klohnen, E. C., & Bera, S. (1998). Behavioral and experiential patterns of avoidantly and securely attached women across adulthood: A 31-year longitudinal perspective. *Journal of Personality and Social Psychology, 74*(1), 211–223.

Kobak, R. R., & Sceery, A. (1988). Attachment in late adolescence: Working models, affect regulation, and representation of self and others. *Child Development, 59,* 135–146.

Kochanska, G. (2001). Emotional development in children with different attachment histories: The first three years. *Child Development, 72*(2), 474–490.

Kohut, H. (1984). *How does analysis cure?* Chicago: University of Chicago Press.

Kotler, T. (1985). Security and autonomy within marriage. *Human Relations, 38,* 299–321.

Kuhn, T. S. (1962). *The structure of scientific revolutions.* Chicago: University of Chicago Press, 1970.

Kuzawa, C. W., Gettler, L. T., Muller, M. N., McDade, T. W., & Feranil, A. B. (2009). Fatherhood, pairbonding, and testosterone in the Philippines. *Hormones and Behavior, 56,* 429–435.

Kuzawa, C. W., Gettler, L. T., Huang, Y., & McDade, T. W. (2010). Mothers have lower testosterone than non-mothers: Evidence from the Philippines. *Hormones and Behavior, 4–5,* 441–447.

Lacan, J. (1960). The subversion of the subject and the dialectic of desire in the Freudian unconscious. In B. Fink (Trans.), *Ecrits* (pp. 671–702). New York: Norton, 2006.

Lakatos, I. (1970). Falsification and the methodology of scientific research programmes. In I. Lakatos & A. Musgrave (Eds.), *Criticism and the growth of knowledge* (pp. 91–196). Cambridge, UK: Cambridge University Press.

Lakatos, I. (1978). *The methodology of scientific research programs: Vol. 1. Philosophical papers.* Cambridge, UK: Cambridge University Press.

Lane, H. (1928). *Talks to parents and teachers.* London: Allen & Unwin.

Latchaw, A. (2010). The relationship between attachment style and degree of unresolved Oedipal conflicts (doctoral dissertation, Adelphi University, The Institute of Advanced Psychological Studies). *ProQuest Dissertations and Theses,* Publication No. 3431571.

Lessard, J. C., & Moretti, M. M. (1998). Suicidal ideation in an adolescent clinical sample: Attachment patterns and clinical implications. *Journal of Adolescence, 21*(4), 383–395.

Levy, K., Beeney, J., & Temes, C. (2011). Attachment and its vicissitudes in borderline personality disorder. *Current Psychiatry Reports, 13*(1), 50–59.

Levy, K. N., & Kelly, K. M. (2010). Sex differences in jealousy: A contribution from attachment theory. *Psychological Science, 21,* 168–173.

Levy, K. N., Meehan, K. B., Kelly, K. M., Reynoso, J. S., Weber, M., Clarkin, J. F., et al. (2006). Change in attachment patterns and reflective function in a randomized control trial of transference-focused psychotherapy for borderline personality disorder. *Journal of Consulting and Clinical Psychology, 74*(6), 1027–1040.

Lewis, M., Feiring, C., McGuffog, C., & Jaskir, J. (1984). Predicting psychopathology in six-year-olds from early social relations. *Child Development, 55,* 123–136.

Lewis, M., Feiring, C., & Rosenthal, S. (2000). Attachment over time. *Child Development, 71*(3), 707–720.

Lieberman, A. F. (1999). Negative maternal attributions: Effects on toddler's sense of self. *Psychoanalytic Inquiry, 19*, 737–756.

Lieberman, A. F., Weston, D. R., & Pawl, J. H. (1991). Preventive intervention and outcome with anxiously attached dyads. *Child Development, 62*, 199–209.

Liebowitz, M. R. (1983). *The chemistry of love*. Boston: Little, Brown.

Lindzey, G. (1967). Some remarks concerning incest, the incest taboo, and psychoanalytic theory. *American Psychologist, 22*, 1051–1059.

Lorenz, K. (1935). The companion in the bird's world: The fellow-member of the species as releasing factor of social behavior. *Journal für Ornithologie Beiblatt* (Leipzig), *83*, 137–213.

Lyons-Ruth, K. (1996). Attachment relationships among children with aggressive behavior problems: The role of disorganized early attachment patterns. *Journal of Consulting and Clinical Psychology, 64*(1), 64–73.

Lyons-Ruth, K., Bronfman, E., & Parsons, E. (1999). Atypical attachment in infancy and early childhood among children at developmental risk: Part IV. Maternal frightened, frightening, or atypical behavior and disorganized infant attachment patterns. In J. Vondra & D. Barnett (Eds.), Atypical patterns of infant attachment: Theory, research, and current directions. *Monographs of the Society for Research in Child Development, 64*(3), 67–96.

Lyons-Ruth, K., Connell, D., Grunebaum, H., & Botein, D. (1990). Infants at social risk: Maternal depression and family support services as mediators of infant development and security of attachment. *Child Development, 61*, 85–98.

Lyons-Ruth, K., & Jacobvitz, D. (2008). Attachment disorganization: Genetic factors, parenting context, and developmental transformation from infancy to adulthood. In J. Cassidy & P. R. Shaver (Eds.), *Handbook of attachment: Theory, research, and clinical applications* (2nd ed., pp. 667–697). New York: Guilford Press.

Mace, C., & Margison, F. (1997). Attachment and psychotherapy: An overview. *British Journal of Medical Psychology, 70*, 209–215.

MacKinnon, D. W., & Dukes, W. F. (1964). Repression. In L. Postman (Ed.), *Psychology in the Making* (pp. 662–744). New York: Knopf.

Madigan, S., Goldberg, S., Moran, G., & Pederson, D. R. (2004). Naïve observers' perceptions of family drawings by 7-year-olds with disorganized attachment histories. *Attachment and Human Development, 6*(3), 223–239.

Madigan, S., Moran, G., Schuengel, C., Pederson, D., & Otten, R. (2007). Unresolved maternal attachment representations, disrupted maternal behavior and disorganized attachment in infancy: Links to toddler behavior problems. *Journal of Child Psychology and Psychiatry and Allied Disciplines, 48*(10), 1042–1050.

Mahler, M. S., Bergman, A., & Pine, F. (1975). *The psychological birth of the human infant: Symbiosis and individuation*. New York: Basic Books.

Mahler, M. S. (1968). *On human symbiosis and the vicissitudes of individuation*. New York: International Universities Press.

Main, M. (1991). Metacognitive knowledge, metacognitive monitoring, and singular (coherent) versus multiple (incoherent) models of attachment: Findings and directions for future research. In C. M. Parkes, J. Stevenson-Hinde, & P. Marris (Eds.), *Attachment across the life cycle* (pp. 127–159). London: Routledge.

Main, M., & Cassidy, J. (1988). Categories of response to reunion with the parent at age 6: Predictable from infant attachment classifications and stable over a 1-month period. *Developmental Psychology, 24,* 415–426.

Main, M., & Goldwyn, R. (1998). *Adult attachment scoring and classification system.* Unpublished scoring manual, Department of Psychology, University of California, Berkeley.

Main, M., & Hesse, E. (1990). Parents' unresolved traumatic experiences are related to infant disorganized attachment status: Is frightened and/or frightening parental behavior the linking mechanism? In M. T. Greenberg, D. Cicchetti, & E. M. Cummings (Eds.), *Attachment in the preschool years: Theory, research, and intervention* (pp. 161–182). Chicago: University of Chicago Press.

Main, M., & Hesse, E. (1995). *Frightening, frightened, timid/deferential, dissociated, or disorganized behavior on the part of the parent: Coding system* (2nd ed.). Unpublished manual, University of California, Berkeley.

Main, M., Kaplan, N., & Cassidy, J. (1985). Security in infancy, childhood, and adulthood: A move to the level of representation. In I. Bretherton & E. Waters (Eds.), Growing points in attachment theory and research. *Monographs of the Society for Research in Child Development, 50*(1–2, Serial No. 209), 60–106.

Main, M., & Solomon, J. (1990). Procedures for identifying infants as disorganized/disoriented during the Ainsworth Strange Situation. In M. T. Greenberg, D. Cicchetti, & E. M. Cummings (Eds.), *Attachment in the preschool years: Theory, research, and intervention* (pp. 121–160). Chicago: University of Chicago Press.

Main, M., & Weston, D. R. (1981). The quality of the toddler's relationship to mother and to father: Related to conflict behavior and the readiness to establish new relationships. *Child Development, 52*(3), 932–940.

Mallinckrodt, B., Gantt, D. L., & Coble, H. M. (1995). Attachment patterns in the psychotherapy relationship: Development of the Client Attachment to Therapist Scale. *Journal of Counseling Psychology, 42,* 307–317.

Mallinckrodt, B., Porter, M. J., & Kivligham, D. M., Jr. (2005). Client attachment to therapist and depth of in-session exploration and object relations in brief psychotherapy. *Psychotherapy: Therapy, Research, Practice, Training, 42,* 85–100.

Manassis, K., Bradley, S., Goldberg, S., Hood, J., & Swinson, R. P. (1994). Attachment in mothers with anxiety disorders and their children. *Journal of the American Academy of Child and Adolescent Psychiatry, 33,* 1106–1113.

Marazziti, D., Dell'Osso, B., Baroni, S., Mungai, F., Catena, M., & Rucci, P. (2006). A relationship between oxytocin and anxiety of romantic attachment. *Clinical Practice and Epidemiology in Mental Health, 2*(28).

Marvin, R. S. (1977). An ethological-cognitive model for the attenuation of mother–infant attachment behavior. In T. M. Alloway, L. Krames, & P. Pliner (Eds.), *Advances in the study of communication and affect: Vol. 3. The development of social attachments* (pp. 25–60). New York: Plenum Press.

Marvin, R. S., Cooper, G., Hoffman, K., & Powell, B. (2002). The Circle of Security project: Attachment-based intervention with caregiver–preschool child dyads. *Attachment and Human Development, 4*, 107–124.

Masterson, J. F., & Rinsley, D. E. (1975). The borderline syndrome: The role of the mother in the genesis and psychic structure of the borderline personality. *International Journal of Psychoanalysis, 56*, 163–177.

Matas, L., Arend, R. A., & Sroufe, L. A. (1978). Continuity of adaptation in the second year: The relationship between quality of attachment and later competence. *Child Development, 49*, 547–556.

Maunder, R. G., & Hunter, J. J. (2001). Attachment and psychosomatic medicine: Developmental contributions to stress and disease. *Psychosomatic Medicine, 63*(4), 556–567.

Maunder, R. G., & Hunter, J. J. (2008). Attachment relationships as determinants of physical health. *Journal of the American Academy of Psychoanalysis and Dynamic Psychiatry, 36*(1), 11–32.

McBride, C., Atkinson, L., Quilty, L. C., & Bagby, R. (2006). Attachment as moderator of treatment outcome in major depression: A randomized control trial of interpersonal psychotherapy versus cognitive behavior therapy. *Journal of Consulting and Clinical Psychology, 74*(6), 1041–1054.

Millon, T. (1983). *Millon Clinical Multiaxial Inventory.* Minneapolis, MN: National Computer Systems.

Mitchell, S. A. (1988). *Relational concepts in psychoanalysis: An integration.* Cambridge, MA: Harvard University Press.

Mitchell, S. A. (1993). Aggression and the endangered self. *Psychoanalytic Quarterly, 62*, 351–382.

Mitchell, S. A. (1998). The analyst's knowledge and authority. *Psychoanalytic Quarterly, 67*, 1–31.

Mitchell, S. A. (2000). *Relationality: From attachment to intersubjectivity.* Hillsdale, NJ: Analytic Press.

Mitchell, S. A. (2002). *Can love last?: The fate of romance over time.* New York: Norton.

Mohr, J. J., Gelso, C. J., & Hill, C. E. (2005). Client and counselor trainee attachment as predictors of session evaluation and countertransference behavior in first counseling sessions. *Journal of Counseling Psychology, 52*, 298–309.

Morehead, D. (1999). Oedipus, Darwin, and Freud: One big, happy family? *Psychoanalytic Quarterly, 68*(3), 347–375.

Moriceau, S., & Sullivan, R. M. (2006). Maternal presence serves as a switch between learning, fear, and attraction in infancy. *Nature Neuroscience, 9*(8), 1004–1006.

Moss, E., & Rousseau, D. (1998). Correlates of attachment at school age: Maternal reported stress, mother–child interaction and behavior problems. *Child Development, 69*(5), 1390.

Moss, E., St-Laurent, D., & Parent, S. (1999). Disorganized attachment and developmental risk at school age. In J. Solomon & C. George (Eds.), *Attachment disorganization* (pp. 160–186). New York: Guilford Press.

Nada-Raja, S., McGee, R., & Stanton, W. R. (1992). Perceived attachment to parents and peers and psychological well-being in adolescence. *Journal of Youth and Adolescence, 21*, 471–485.

Newcombe, N., & Lerner, J. C. (1982). Britain between the wars: The historical context of Bowlby's theory of attachment. *Psychiatry, 45*(1), 1–12.

Obegi, J. H., & Berant, E. (Eds.). (2009). *Attachment theory and research in clinical work with adults*. New York: Guilford Press.

Ogawa, J., Sroufe, L., Weinfield, N., Carlson, E., & Egeland, B. (1997). Development and the fragmented self: Longitudinal study of dissociative symptomatology in a nonclinical sample. *Development and Psychopathology, 9*(4), 855–879.

Ogden, T. (1982). *Projective identification and therapeutic technique*. New York: Jason Aronson.

O'Shea-Lauber, K. A. (2000). The physiological cost of repressive style and adult attachment style (Doctoral dissertation, Adelphi University, The Institute of Advanced Psychological Studies). *ProQuest Dissertations and Theses*, Publication No. 9988057.

Owens, G., Crowell, J. A., Pan, H., & Treboux, D. (1995). The prototype hypothesis and the origins of attachment working models: Adult relationships with parents and romantic partners. *Monographs of the Society for Research in Child Development, 60*(2–3), 216–233.

Parens, H. (1979). *The development of aggression in early childhood*. New York: Jason Aronson.

Parish, M., & Eagle, M. N. (2003). Attachment to the therapist. *Psychoanalytic Psychology, 20*(2), 271–286.

Parker, J. G., & Asher, S. R. (1987). Peer relations and later personal adjustment: Are low-accepted children at risk? *Psychological Bulletin, 12*, 357–389.

Passman, R. H., & Erck, T. W. (1977, March). *Visual presentation of mothers for facilitating play in children: The affects of silent films of mothers*. Paper presented at the meeting of Society for Research in Child Development, New Orleans, LA.

Passman, R. H., & Longeway, K. P. (1982). The role of vision in maternal attachment: Giving 2-year-olds a photograph of their mother during separation. *Developmental Psychology, 18*(4), 530–533.

Patrick, M., Hobson, P., Castle, D., Howard, R., & Maughan, B. (1994). Personality disorder and the mental representation of early social experience. *Development and Psychopathology, 6*, 375–388.

Pearson, J. L., Cohn, D. A., Cowan, P. A., & Cowan, C. (1994). Earned- and continuous-security in adult attachment: Relation to depressive symptomatology and parenting style. *Development and Psychopathology, 6*(2), 359–373.

Pederson, D. R., Moran, G., Sitco, C., Campbell, K., Ghesquire, K., & Acton, H. (1990). Maternal sensitivity and the security of infant–mother attachment: A Q-sort study. *Child Development, 61*, 1974–1983.

Polan, J. H., & Hofer, M. A. (2008). Psychobiological origins of infant attachment and its role in development. In J. Cassidy & P. R. Shaver (Eds.), *Handbook of attachment: Theory, research, and clinical applications* (2nd ed., pp. 158–172). New York: Guilford Press.

Pollet, T. V., van der Meij, L., Cobey, K. D., & Buunk, A. P. (2011). Testosterone levels and their associations with lifetime number of opposite sex partners and remarriage in a large sample of American elderly men and women. *Hormones and Behavior, 60*, 72–77.

Posada, G., Gao, Y., Wu, F., Posada, R., Tascon, M., Schöelmerich, A., et al. (1995). The secure-base phenomenon across cultures: Children's behavior, mothers' preferences, and experts' concepts. *Monographs of the Society for Research in Child Development, 60*(2–3), 27–48.

Powers, S. I., Pietromonaco, P. R., Gunlicks, M., & Sayer, A. (2006). Dating couples' attachment styles and patterns of cortisol reactivity and recovery in response to a relationship conflict. *Journal of Personality and Social Psychology, 90*(4), 613–628.

Rajecki D. W., Lamb M. E., & Obmascher, P. (1978). Toward a general theory of infantile attachment: A comparative review of aspects of the social bond. *Behavioral and Brain Sciences, 3*, 417–464.

Rapaport, D. (1967). *Collected papers* (M. M. Gill, Ed.). New York: Basic Books.

Raval, V., Goldberg, S., Atkinson, L., Benoit, D., Myhal, N., Poulton, L., et al. (2001). Maternal attachment, maternal responsiveness and infant attachment. *Infant Behavior and Development, 24*(3), 281–304.

Renken, B., Egeland, B., Marvinney, D., Mangelshdof, S., & Sroufe, L. A. (1989). Early childhood antecedents of aggression and passive withdrawal in early elementary school. *Journal of Personality, 57*, 257–281.

Rholes, W. S., Simpson, J. A., & Orina, M. M. (1999). Attachment and anger in an anxiety-provoking situation. *Journal of Personality and Social Psychology, 76*, 940–957.

Ribble, M. (1943). *The rights of infants*. New York: Columbia University Press.

Riggs, S. A., Paulson, A., Tunnell, E., Sahl, G., Atkison, H., & Ross, C. A. (2007). Attachment, personality, and psychopathology among adult inpatients: Self-reported romantic attachment style versus Adult Attachment Interview states of mind. *Development and Psychopathology, 19*, 263–291.

Rivière, J. (1927). Contribution to symposium on child analysis. *International Journal of Psycho-Analysis, 8*, 339–391.

Robertson, J. (1962). *Hospitals and children: A parent's eye view: A review of letters from parents to The Observer and the BBC*. London: Victor Gollancz.

Roisman, G. I. (2007). The psychophysiology of adult attachment relationships: Autonomic reactivity in marital and premarital interactions. *Developmental Psychology, 43*(1), 39–53.

Roisman, G. I., Fortuna, K., & Holland, A. (2006). An experimental manipulation of retrospectively defined earned and continuous attachment security. *Child Development, 77*(1), 59–71.

Roisman, G. I., & Fraley, R. (2006). The limits of genetic influence: A behavior-genetic analysis of infant–caregiver relationship quality and temperament. *Child Development, 77*(6), 1656–1667.

Roisman, G. I., Holland, A., Fortuna, K., Fraley, R., Clausell, E., & Clarke, A. (2007). The Adult Attachment Interview and self-reports of attachment style:

An empirical rapprochement. *Journal of Personality and Social Psychology*, 92(4), 678–697.

Roisman, G. I., Padrón, E., Sroufe, L., & Egeland, B. (2002). Earned-secure attachment status in retrospect and prospect. *Child Development*, 73(4), 1204–1219.

Roisman, G. I., Tsai, J. L., & Chiang, K. (2004). The emotional integration of childhood experience: Physiological, facial expressive, and self-reported emotional response during the Adult Attachment Interview. *Developmental Psychology*, 40(5), 776–789.

Rosenstein, D. S., & Horowitz, H. A. (1996). Adolescent attachment and psychopathology. *Journal of Consulting and Clinical Psychology*, 64, 244–253.

Rosenzweig, S. (1934). An experimental study of memory in relation to the theory of repression. *British Journal of Psychology*, 24, 247–265.

Rubino, G., Barker, C., Roth, T., & Featon, R. M. P. (2000). Therapist empathy and depth of interpretation in response to potential alliance ruptures: The role of therapist and patient attachment styles. *Psychotherapy Research*, 10, 408–420.

Rutter, M. (1976). Parent–child separation: Psychological effects on the children. In A. M. Clarke & A. D. B. Clarke (Eds.), *Early experience: Myth and evidence* (pp. 153–186). New York: Free Press.

Rutter, M., Quinton, D., & Hill, J. (1990). Adult outcome of institution-reared children: Males and females compared. In L. Robbins & M. Rutter (Eds.), *Straight and deviant pathways from childhood to adulthood* (pp. 135–157). Cambridge, UK: Cambridge University Press.

Ryle, A. (1990). *Cognitive analytic therapy: Active participation in change*. Chichester, UK: Wiley.

Sauer, E. M., Lopez, F. G., & Gormley, B. (2003). Respective contributions of therapist and client adult attachment orientations to the development of the early working alliance: A preliminary growth modeling study. *Psychotherapy Research*, 13(3), 371–382.

Scarf, M. (1976). *Body, mind, behavior*. Washington, DC: New Republic.

Schachter, J. (2002). *Transference: Shibboleth or albatross?* New York: Analytic Press.

Schanberg, S., & Kuhn, C. (1980). Maternal deprivation: An animal model of psychosocial dwarfism. In E. Usdin, T. Sourks, & M. Youdin (Eds.), *Enzymes and neurotransmitters in mental disease* (pp. 373–393). Chichester, UK: Wiley.

Schank, R. C., & Abelson, R. D. (1982). *Dynamic memory: A theory of reminding and learning in computers and people*. New York: Cambridge University Press.

Schauenburg, H. B., Buchheim, A., Beckh, T. N., Brenk-Franz, K., Leichsenring, F., Strack, M., et al. (2010). The influence of psychodynamically oriented therapists' attachment representations on outcome and alliance in inpatient psychotherapy. *Psychotherapy Research*, 20(2), 192–202.

Schneider-Rosen, K. (1990). The devopmental reorganization of attachment relationships: Guidelines for classification beyond infancy. In M. P. Greenberg,

D. Cicchetti, & E. M. Cummings (Eds.), *Attachment in the preschool years*. (pp. 185–220). Chicago: University of Chicago Press.

Schuengel, C., Bakermans-Kranenburg, M. J., & van IJzendoorn, M. H. (1999). Frightening maternal behavior linking unresolved loss and disorganized attachment. *Journal of Consulting and Clinical Psychology, 67*, 54–63.

Schwartz, G. E. (1990). Psychophysiology of repression and health: A systems approach. In J. L. Singer (Ed.), *Repression and dissociation* (pp. 405–434). Chicago: University of Chicago Press.

Segal, H. (1964). *Introduction to the work of Melanie Klein*. New York: Basic Books.

Shaver, P. R. (2011, June 8–11). *Attachment and research*. Paper presented at panel at the spring meeting of the American Psychoanalytic Association, San Francisco.

Shaw, D. S., Keenan, K., Vondra, J. I., Delliquadri, E., & Giovannelli, J. (1997). Antecedents of preschool children's internalizing problems: A longitudinal study of low-income families. *Journal of the American Academy of Child and Adolescent Psychiatry, 36*, 1760–1767.

Shedler, J., Mayman, M., & Manis, M. (1993). The illusion of mental health. *American Psychologist, 48*(11), 1117–1131.

Shepher, J. (1971). Mate selection among second generation kibbutz adolescents and adults: Incest avoidance and negative imprinting. *Archives of Sexual Behavior, 1*, 293–307.

Sherwin, B. B., & Gelfand, M. M. (1987). The role of androgen in the maintenance of sexual functioning in oophorectomized women. *Psychosomatic Medicine, 49*, 397–409.

Sherwin, B. B., Gelfand, M. M., & Brender, W. (1985). Androgen enhances sexual motivation in females: A prospective, crossover study of sex steroid administration in the surgical menopause. *Psychosomatic Medicine, 47*, 339–351.

Shor, E., & Simchai, D. (2009). Incest avoidance, the incest taboo, and social cohesion: Revisiting Westermarck and the case of the Israeli kibbutzim. *American Journal of Sociology, 114*(6), 1803–1842.

Silverman, D. K. (1991). Attachment patterns and Freudian theory: An integrative proposal. *Psychoanalytic Psychology, 8*, 169–175.

Slade, A. (1999). Attachment theory and research: Implications for the theory and practice of individual psychotherapy with adults. In J. Cassidy & P. R. Shaver (Eds.), *Handbook of attachment: Theory, research, and clinical applications* (pp. 575–594). New York: Guilford Press.

Slade, A., & Sadler, L.S. (November 3, 2012). *Minding the baby: Enhancing mentalization in traumatized mothers and their children*. Keynote presentation, Association for Infant Mental Health UK, London, England.

Slade, A. (2008). The implications of attachment theory and research for adult psychotherapy: Research and clinical perspectives. In J. Cassidy & P. R. Shaver (Eds.), *Handbook of attachment: Theory, research, and clinical applications* (2nd ed., pp. 762–782). New York: Guilford Press.

Slade, A., Sadler, L., & Mayes, L. C. (2005). Minding the baby: Enhancing parental reflective functioning in a nursing/mental health home visiting program.

In L. Berlin, Y. Ziv, L. Amaya-Jackson, & M. T. Greenberg (Eds.), *Enhancing early attachments: Theory, research, intervention, and policy* (pp. 152–177). New York: Guilford Press.

Sloan, E. P., Maunder, R. G., Hunter, J. J., & Moldofsky, H. (2007). Insecure attachment is associated with the α-EEG anomaly during sleep. *BioPsycho-Social Medicine, 1*(20), 1–6.

Solomon, J., & George, C. (1999). The measurement of attachment security in infancy and childhood. In J. Cassidy & P. R. Shaver (Eds.), *Handbook of attachment: Theory, research, and clinical applications* (pp. 287–316). New York: Guilford Press.

Solomon, J., George, C., & De Jong, A. (1995). Children classified as controlling at age six: Evidence of disorganized representational strategies and aggression at home and at school. *Development and Psychopathology, 7*, 447–463.

Sorce, J. F., & Emde, R. N. (1981). Mother's presence is not enough: Effect of emotional availability on infant exploration. *Developmental Psychology, 17*(6), 737–745.

Spelke, E. S. (1990). Principles of object perception. *Cognitive Science: A Multidisciplinary Journal, 14*(1), 29–56.

Spence, D. P. (1982). *Narrative truth and historical truth.* New York: Norton.

Spitz, R. A. (1965). *The first year of life.* New York: International Universities Press.

Sroufe, L. A. (1983). Infant–caregiver attachment and patterns of adaptation in preschool: The roots of maladaptation and competence. In M. Perlmutter (Ed.), *Minnesota Symposium in Child Psychology* (Vol. 16, pp. 41– 83). Hillsdale, NJ: Erlbaum.

Sroufe, L. A. (1985). Attachment classification from the perspective of infant–caregiver relationships and infant temperament. *Child Development, 56*(1), 1–14.

Sroufe, L. A., Egeland, B., Carlson, E., & Collins, W. A. (2005a). *The development of the person: The Minnesota study of risk and adaptation from birth to adulthood.* New York: Guilford Press.

Sroufe, L. A., Egeland, B., Carlson, E., & Collins, W. A. (2005b). Placing early attachment experiences in developmental context. In K. E. Grossmann, K. Grossmann, & E. Waters (Eds.), *Attachment from infancy to adulthood: The major longitudinal studies* (pp. 48–70). New York: Guilford Press.

Sroufe, L. A., & Fleeson, J. (1986). Attachment and the construction of relationships. In W. W. Hartup & Z. Rubin (Eds.), *Relationships and development* (pp. 36–54). Hillsdale, NJ: Erlbaum.

Sroufe, L. A., Schork, E., Motti, E., Lawroski, N., & LaFreniere, P. (1984). The role of affect in social competence. In C. Izard, G. Kagan, & R. Zajonc (Eds.), *Emotion, cognition and behavior* (pp. 289–319). New York: Plenum Press.

Sroufe, L. A., & Waters, E. (1977). Heart rate as a convergent measure in clinical and developmental research. *Merrill-Palmer Quarterly, 23*, 3–27.

Sterba, R. F. (1934). The fate of the ego in analytic therapy. *International Journal of Psychoanalysis, 115*, 117–126.

Stern, D. N. (1985). *The interpersonal world of the human infant*. New York: Basic Books.

Sternberg, K. J., Lamb, M. E., Greenbaum, C., Cicchetti, D., Dawud, S., Cortes, R. M., et al. (1993). Effects of intimate partner violence on children's behavior problems and depression. *Developmental Psychology, 29*, 44–52.

Stich, S. (1983). *From folk psychology to cognitive science: The case against belief*. Cambridge, MA: MIT Press.

Stoff, J., & Eagle, M. (1971). Reported strategies, presentation rate and verbal ability: Their relationship to free recall. *Journal of Experimental Psychology, 87*, 423–428.

Stolorow, R. D., Atwood, G. E., & Orange, D. M. (2002). *Worlds of experience*. New York: Basic Books.

Stovall-McClough, K. C., & Cloitre, M. (2006). Unresolved attachment and PTSD and dissociation in women with childhood abuse histories. *Journal of Consulting and Clinical Psychology, 74*, 219–228.

Stovall-McClough, K. C., Cloitre, M., & McClough, J. F. (2008). Adult attachment and posttraumatic stress disorder in women with histories of childhood abuse. In H. Steele & M. Steele (Eds.), *Clinical applications of the Adult Attachment Interview* (pp. 320–340). New York: Guilford Press.

Strachey, J. (1937). Editor's note to analysis terminable and interminable. *Standard Edition*, Vol. 23, p. 211. London: Hogarth Press, 1964.

Strathearn, L., Fonagy, P., Amico, J., & Montague, P. R. (2009). Adult attachment predicts maternal brain and oxytocin response to infant cues. *Neuropsychopharmacology, 34*, 2655–2666.

Stroebe, W., Stroebe, M., Abakoumkin, G., & Schut, H. (1996). The role of loneliness and social support in adjustment to loss: A test of attachment versus stress theory. *Journal of Personality and Social Psychology, 70*(6), 1241–1249.

Strupp, H., & Binder, J. L. (1984). *Psychotherapy in a new key*. New York: Basic Books.

Sugarman, A. (2006). Mentalization, insightfulness, and therapeutic action: The importance of mental organization. *International Journal of Psychoanalysis, 87*, 965–987.

Sullivan, H. S. (1953). *Conceptions of modern psychiatry*. New York: Norton.

Sullivan, R. M., & Lasley, E. N. (2010, September/October). Fear in love: Attachment, abuse, and the developing brain. *Cerebrum*. Retrieved from *www.dana.org/news/cerebrum/detail.aspx?id=28926*.

Sullivan, R. M., Landers, M., Yeaman, B., & Wilson, D. A. (2000). Good memories of bad events in infancy: Ontogeny of conditioned fear and the amygdala. *Nature, 407*, 38–39.

Suttie, I. D. (1935). *The origins of love and hate*. London: Free Association Books, 1988.

Symons, D. (1979). *The evolution of human sexuality*. New York: Oxford University Press.

Talmon, Y. (1964). Mate selection in collective settlements. *American Sociological Review, 29*, 491–508.

Thiessen, D. D., & Gregg, B. (1980). Human assortative mating and genetic equilibrium: An evolutionary perspective. *Ethology and Sociobiology, 1,* 111–140.

Thompson. A. P. (1983). Extramarital sex: A review of the research literature. *Journal of Sex Research, 19,* 1–22.

Tierney, J. (2003, September 28). The struggle for Iraq: Traditions; Iraqi family ties complicate American efforts for change. *The New York Times.*

Tini, M., Corcoran, D., Rodriques-Doolabh, L., & Waters, E. (2003). *Maternal attachment scripts and infant secure base behavior.* Poster presented at the biennial meeting of the Society for Research in Child Development, Tampa, FL.

Tolman, E. C. (1948). Cognitive maps in rats and men. *Psychology Review, 55,* 189–208.

Tops, M., Van Peer, J. M., Korf, J., Wijers, A. A., & Tucker, D. M. (2007). Anxiety, cortisol and attachment predict plasma oxytocin levels in healthy females. *Psychophysiology, 44*(3), 444–449.

Toth, S. L., Cicchetti, D., Macfie, J., & Emde, R. N. (1997). Representations of self and other in the narratives of neglected, physically abused, and sexually abused pre-schoolers. *Development and Psychopathology, 9,* 781–796.

Toth, S. L., Cicchetti, D., Macfie, J., Rogosch, F. A., & Maughan, A. (2000). Narrative representation of moral-affiliative and conflictual themes and behavior problems in maltreated pre-schoolers. *Journal of Clinical Child Psychology, 29,* 307–318.

Toth, S. L., Manly, J. T., & Cicchetti, D. (1992). Child maltreatment and vulnerability to depression. *Development and Psychopathology, 4,* 97–112.

Toth, S. L., Rogosch, F. A., Manly, J., & Cicchetti, D. (2006). The efficacy of toddler–parent psychotherapy to reorganize attachment in the young offspring of mothers with major depressive disorder: A randomized preventive trial. *Journal of Consulting and Clinical Psychology, 74*(6), 1006–1016.

Trivers, R. L. (1971). The evolution of reciprocal altruism. *Quarterly Review of Biology, 46,* 35–57.

Troisi, A., D'Argenio, A., Peracchio, F., & Petti, P. (2001). Insecure attachment and alexithymia in young men with mood symptoms. *Journal of Nervous and Mental Disease, 189*(5), 311–316.

Troy, M., & Sroufe, L. (1987). Victimization among preschoolers: Role of attachment relationship history. *Journal of the American Academy of Child and Adolescent Psychiatry, 26,* 166–172.

Tyrrell, C. L., Dozier, M., & Teague, G. B. (1999). Effective treatment relationships for persons with serious psychiatric disorders: The importance of attachment states of mind. *Journal of Consulting and Clinical Psychology, 67*(5), 725–733.

Vaillant, G. E. (1971). Theoretical hierarchy of adaptive ego mechanisms: 30-year follow-up of 30 men selected for psychological health. *Archives of General Psychiatry, 33,* 535–545.

Vaillant, G. E. (1975). Natural history of male psychological health, III: Empirical dimensions of mental health. *Archives of General Psychiatry, 32,* 420–426.

Vaillant, G. E. (1976). Natural history of male psychological health, IV: The relation of choice of ego mechanisms of defense to adult adjustment. *Archives of General Psychiatry, 33,* 535–545.

van den Boom, D. C. (1989). Neonatal irritability and the development of attachment. In G. A. Kohnstamm & J. E. Bates (Eds.), *Temperament in childhood* (pp. 299–318). Oxford, UK: Wiley.

van den Boom, D. C. (1994). The influence of temperament and mothering on attachment and exploration: An experimental manipulation of sensitive responsiveness among lower-class mothers with irritable infants. *Child Development, 65*(5), 1457–1477.

van den Boom, D. C. (1995). Do first-year intervention effects endure?: Follow-up during toddlerhood of a sample of Dutch irritable infants. *Child Development, 66*(6), 1798–1816.

van der Horst, F. P. (2011). *John Bowlby—From psychoanalysis to ethology: Unraveling the roots of attachment theory.* New York: Wiley Online Library.

van IJzendoorn, M. H. (1995). Adult attachment representations, parental responsiveness, and infant attachment: A meta-analysis on the predictive validity of the Adult Attachment Interview. *Psychological Bulletin, 117*(3), 387–403.

van IJzendoorn, M. H., & Bakermans-Kranenburg, M. J. (2006). DRD4 7-repeat polymorphism moderates the association between unresolved loss or trauma and infant disorganization. *Attachment and Human Development, 8,* 291–307.

van IJzendoorn, M. H., Juffer, F., & Duyvesteyn, M. G. C. (1995). Breaking the intergenerational cycle of insecure attachment: A review of the effects of attachment-based interventions on maternal sensitivity and infant security. *Journal of Child Psychology and Psychiatry, 36,* 225–248.

van IJzendoorn, M. H., Moran, G., Belsky, J., Pederson, D., Bakermans-Kranenburg, M., & Kneppers, K. (2000). The similarity of siblings' attachments to their mother. *Child Development, 71*(4), 1086–1098.

Waller, E., Scheidt, C. E., & Hartmann, A. (2004). Attachment representation and illness behavior in somatoform disorders. *Journal of Neurons and Mental Disease, 192*(3), 200–209.

Wallin, D. (2007). *Attachment in psychotherapy.* New York: Guilford Press.

Wampler, K. S., Riggs, B., & Kimball, T. G. (2004). Observing Attachment Behavior in Couples: The Adult Attachment Behavior Q-Set (AABQ). *Family Process, 43*(3), 315–335.

Ward, A., Ramsay, R., Turnbull, S., Steele, M., Steele, H., & Treasure, J. (2001). Attachment in anorexia nervosa: A transgenerational perspective. *British Journal of Medical Psychology, 74,* 497–505.

Ward, M. J., Lee, S. S., & Polan, H. J. (2006). Attachment and psychopathology in a community sample. *Attachment and Human Development, 8,* 327–340.

Waring, E. M., Tillman, M. P., Frelick, L., Russell, L., & Weisz, G. (1980). Concepts of intimacy in the general population. *Journal of Neurons and Mental Disease, 168*(8), 471–474.

Warren, S. L., Huston, L., Egeland, B., & Sroufe, L. A. (1997). Child and adolescent anxiety disorders and early attachment. *Journal of the American Academy of Child and Adolescent Psychiatry, 36,* 637–644.

Wartner, U. G., Grossmann, K., Fremmer-Bombik, E., & Suess, G. (1994). Attachment patterns at age six in south Germany: Predictability from infancy and implications for preschool behavior. *Child Development, 65*(4), 1014–1027.

Waters, E. (1995). Appendix A: The Attachment Q-Set (Version 3.0). *Monographs of the Society for Research in Child Development, 60*(2–3), 234–246.

Waters, E. (2009, March). *The central role of the secure base concept in Bowlby–Ainsworth attachment theory.* Invited talk to the New York Psychoanalytic Society and Institute

Waters, E., Crowell, J., Elliot, M., Corcoran, D., & Treboux, D. (2002). Bowlby's secure base theory and social/personality psychology of attachment style: Work(s) in progress. *Attachment and Human Development, 4,* 230–242.

Waters, E., Merrick, S., Treboux, D., Crowell, J., & Albersheim, L. (2000). Attachment security in infancy and early adulthood: A twenty-year longitudinal study. *Child Development, 71*(3), 684–689.

Waters, H., & Rodrigues-Doolabh, L. M. (2001, April). *Are attachment scripts the building blocks of attachment representations?: Narrative assessment of representations and the AAI.* Paper presented at the biennial meeting of the Society for Research in Child Development, Minneapolis, MN.

Waters, H. S., & Waters, E. (2006). The attachment working models concept: Among other things, we build script-like representations of secure base experiences. *Attachment and Human Development, 8*(3), 185–197.

Waters, T. E. A., & Brockmeyer, S. L. (in press). AAI coherence predicts attachment behavior in couple problem solving interactions: Secure base script knowledge helps explain why. *Attachment & Human Development.*

Weisberger, C. (2000, March). Infidelity in dating relationships: Examining the impact of attachment style differences on infidelity. Paper presented at the Annual Southern States Communication Association Meetings, New Orleans, Louisiana.

Weiss, J., & Sampson, H. (1986). *The psychoanalytic process: Theory, clinical observation, and empirical research.* New York: Guilford Press.

Weiss, R. S. (1973). *Loneliness: The experience of emotional and social isolation.* Cambridge, MA: MIT Press.

Weiss, R. S. (1982). Attachment in adult life. In C. M. Parkes & J. Stevenson-Hinde (Eds.), *The place of attachment in human behavior* (pp. 171–184). New York: Basic Books.

West, M., Adam, K., Spreng, S., & Rose, S. (2001). Attachment disorganisation and dissociative symptoms in clinically treated adolescents. *Canadian Journal of Psychiatry, 46,* 627–631.

Westermarck, E. (1891). *The history of human marriage.* London: Macmillan.

Westermarck, E. (1926). *A short history of marriage.* London: Macmillan.

White, K. (2004). Developing a secure-enough base: Teaching psychotherapists in training the relationship between attachment theory and clinical work. *Attachment and Human Development, 6*(2), 117–130.

White, R. W. (1959). Motivations reconsidered: The concept of competence. *Psychological Review, 66*, 297–333.

Whitfield, C. L., Anda, R. F., Dube, S. R., & Felitti, V. J. (2003). Violent childhood experiences and the risk of intimate partner violence in adults: Assessment in a large health maintenance organization. *Journal of Interpersonal Violence, 18*, 166–185.

Widlocher, D. (2002). Primary love and infantile sexuality: An eternal debate. *Infantile sexuality and attachment* (pp. 1–36). London: Karnac Books.

Wingfield, J. C. (1984). Androgens and mating systems: Testosterone-induced polygyny in normally monogamous birds. *The Auk, 101*, 665–671.

Winnicott, D. W. (1953). Transitional objects and transitional phenomena. *International Journal of Psychoanalysis, 34*, 89–97.

Winnicott, D. W. (1965). Ego distortion in terms of true and false self. In *The maturational processes and the facilitating environment* (pp. 140–152). New York: International Universities Press.

Yunger, J. L., Corby, B. C., & Perry, D. G. (2005). Dimensions of attachment in middle childhood. In K. A. Kerns & R. A. Richardson (Eds.). *Attachment in middle childhood* (pp. 89–114). New York: Guilford Press.

Zajonc, R., Adelmann, P., Murphy, S., & Niedenthal, P. (1987). Convergence in the physical appearance of spouses. *Motivation and Emotion, 11*, 335–346.

Zak, P. J., Kurzban, R., & Matzner, W. T. (2005). Oxytocin is associated with human trustworthiness. *Hormones and Behavior, 48*, 522–527.

Zeanah, C. H. (1996). Beyond insecurity: A reconceptualization of attachment disorders in infancy. *Journal of Consulting and Clinical Psychology, 64*, 42–52.

Zeanah, C. H., Smyke, A. T., Koga, S. F., Carlson, E., & the Bucharest Early Intervention Project Care Group. (2005). Attachment in institutionalized and community children in Romania. *Child Development, 76*, 1015–1028.

Index